A GUIDE FOR
THE MODERN PRACTITIONER

KAREN HORNEY
& CHARACTER DISORDER

About the Author

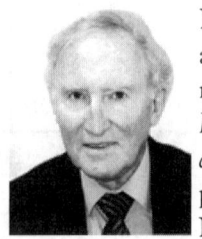

IRVING SOLOMON, PHD, is a psychologist–psychoanalyst and a Diplomate in Clinical Psychology. He has authored numerous papers on psychotherapy and two books, *The Encyclopedia of Evolving Techniques in Dynamic Psychotherapy* and *A Primer of Kleinian Therapy*. He maintains a private practice of psychodynamic therapy in Rockville Centre, New York.

A GUIDE FOR
THE MODERN PRACTITIONER

KAREN HORNEY
& CHARACTER DISORDER

IRVING SOLOMON, PhD

 Springer Publishing Company

Photograph of Irving Solomon taken by Ira Brophy.

Springer Publishing Company, Inc.
11 West 42nd Street
New York, NY 10036

Acquisitions Editor: Lauren Dockett
Production Editor: Jeanne Libby
Cover design by Mimi Flow

06 07 08 09 10 / 5 4 3 2 1

_____

Library of Congress Cataloging-in-Publication Data

Solomon, Irving.
    Karen Horney and character disorder : a guide for the modern
practitioner / Irving Solomon.
        p. cm.
    Includes bibliographical references and index.
    ISBN 0-8261-2995-1 (soft cover)
    1. Horney, Karen, 1885–1952. 2. Psychology, Pathological.
3. Psychoanalysis. I. Title.

RC506.S62 2006
616.89'17—dc22

2005017981

_____

Printed in the United States of America by Sheridan Books, Inc.

For
Sandra; Neil and Patty, Rebecca and Daniel;
Leigh and Tommy, Jackie and T.J.

Contents

Preface

My first contact with Karen Horney's psychoanalytic theory and therapy originated from a surprising source. I had just begun a four year postdoctoral training program in psychotherapy and psychoanalysis at Adelphi University. During the first year the students were required to participate in a course dealing with the basic principles of psychotherapy. The class at that time was taught by Jules Nydes, a much admired instructor, former analysand of the eminent Freudian psychoanalyst, Dr. Theodor Reik. Much to my astonishment Nydes asked us to read the chapter, "The Road of Psychoanalytic Therapy" in Karen Horney's book *Neurosis and Human Growth* (1950a, pp. 333–365). As I began to study the chapter I recalled vaguely that Horney was labeled a NeoFreudian and definitely out of favor with the dominant classical Freudian camp, but I was struck by the finding that her writing was remarkable for its crystal-clear expression. In contrast to the vast majority of psychoanalytic writers of journal papers and books, Horney vigorously wrote better than they in simple, lucid prose about problems of the inner heart in conflict with itself.

She also led me to an elegant, necessary panoramic view of psychotherapy. I liked her recognition that therapy (i.e., in my practice mainly once-per-week sessions) is urgent; that it is, like much of life, fired at us point blank within each session. I sensed her respect for the right of each patient to restore his or her vitality, to take stock of their own capabilities and not hide their strengths because of basic anxiety (i.e., Horney's concept). She, in her chapter, reminded me once more of the significance of Montaigne's wise statement about self-depreciation, namely, that "It is

ix

a malady confined to man, and not seen in any other creature, to hate and despise himself. It is on a par with our vanity to desire to be other than we are."

Much later my admiration for Horney grew even more when I read about her painful, courageous conflict with the self-appointed gurus of the New York Psychoanalytic Society. Horney had gathered as an instructor in the New York Psychoanalytic Institute many students attracted by her clear exposition and the value of her ideas. Nonetheless, she was dismissed form the society by a powerful, rigid, dogmatic inner circle on the spurious, shabby grounds that she was "upsetting" the students. "Upsetting" apparently meant to them, a free and open exchange of different points of view about what makes for an effective psychoanalytic therapy.

At her dismissal Karen stood up ". . . and with great dignity, her head held high, slowly walked out" (Rubins, 1978, p. 240). Accompanied by a number of her supportive colleagues, she and they marched down the street and they sang ". . . Karen's favorite spiritual: 'Go down Moses, way down in Egypt land, Tell old Pharaoh, to let my people go'—the song celebrating the liberation of the Jews from Egyptian tyranny" (Rubins, 1978, p. 240).

Undaunted Horney continued to contribute significantly as a writer, teacher, and founder of the Karen Horney Society and Institute, to the advancement of psychoanalytic therapy. Her major ideas, both theoretical and clinical, that are vital to the understanding and treatment of character pathology are gathered together, explained, and illustrated in this book.

Karen Horney and Character Disorder: A Guide for the Modern Practitioner is intended for every mental health professional who takes on the challenge of treating a patient who has a character disorder, the most pervasive pathology of our time.

Acknowledgments

I want to acknowledge my great debt to my wife, Sandra, who steadfastly encouraged and aided me in the creation of this volume. I wish to acknowledge the expertise of Ms. Dockett, an Editor at the Springer Publishing Company, who asked probing questions and made suggestions that without a doubt improved the quality of this book. I also wish to thank Dr. Macias who graciously permitted me the use of the library facilities at the Karen Horney Institute which provided me with helpful data.

IRVING SOLOMON

1 Introduction

Who is Karen Horney and why are her psychoanalytic ideas so important in today's world of once-per-week dynamic psychotherapy?

A BRIEF SKETCH OF HORNEY'S LIFE

There is a photo on the cover of Bernard J. Paris' fine biography (1994) of Karen Horney, which depicts her seated at a table with a cigarette in her left hand and a drink in her right hand. She is smiling and the effect of her smile and posture conveys a love of life, a capacity for joy and enthusiasm.

Another biographer, Jack Rubins (1978), after extensive interviews with people who knew Horney, concludes that she was a complex personality.

> She needed to encompass and unify many diverse and conflicting traits, apparently with constant struggle. But no one who knew her was unaffected by her; all spoke of her with passion. All agreed that she exerted a strong influence upon them. Her charisma—that most misused and difficult to define of words—was evident. (Rubins, 1978, p. XIV)

Susan Quinn titles her biography (1987) of Karen Horney "A Mind of Her Own," to emphasize what she considers her greatest strength. Horney showed throughout her life an independence of mind and spirit.

She consistently relied on her own experience to test the reality and validity of any view of behavior.

The preceding statements describe Karen Horney as an adult, but what was she like as a child? What were the personalities of her parents and siblings? Where was she born?

Karen Horney (1885–1952) was born in a suburb of Hamburg, Germany. Her father was a commodore with the Hamburg-American shipping line and was generally known as Captain Danielson. His first wife died and he subsequently married Clotilde Van Ronzelen, Karen's mother. Captain Danielson was 18 years her senior.

Karen's father was a stern, religious man who could quote from the bible and would be considered a fundamentalist by today's standards. He apparently had a vile temper, for he would sometimes fling his bible at his wife if he felt she displeased him.

Perhaps because of Karen's father's religious beliefs he favored her older brother, Berndt. Karen's mother, Sonni (her nickname in the family) disputed this favoritism. Sonni was better educated and more sophisticated than her husband and could be more tolerant than he was. Karen had ambivalent feelings toward her father, on the one hand admiring him for his love of life and on the other hand fearing and being intimidated by him. Her father's irascible temper and stern demandingness apparently fostered so much marital tension that Sonni divorced him when Karen was almost 20.

Karen Horney was a fine student. She was goal-oriented, energetically imaginative, intuitive, and intellectually gifted. In medical school she found life exhilarating and liberating. She attacked and assimilated the subject matter with relish and success. She received her medical degree in 1913.

During her medical studies Karen met and married Oskar Horney, who eventually earned a Ph.D. in law, economics, and political science. He occupied an executive position in a major industrial firm and did well financially until his firm fell apart during the inflation of 1933. Ultimately Karen separated from Oskar because she felt he was too lacking in elemental passion, too limited in strength and pride. She craved a stronger man. Karen took their three daughters and moved into a small apartment near Oskar.

During the years of World War I she was analyzed by two major psychoanalytic pioneers, Karl Abraham and Hanns Sachs. She became a psychoanalyst and a faculty member of the Berlin Psychoanalytic Institute.

In 1931, Franz Alexander, director of the Chicago Institute for Psychoanalysis, invited Horney to come to America and accept the position of associate director of his institute. He greatly admired her independent thinking and her clear exposition of ideas. She accepted the invitation and remained in Chicago from 1932 to 1934, relocating to New York when collegian tensions occurred between her and Alexander. There she affiliated with the New York Psychoanalytic Institute, the major medical psychoanalytic training school in the Freudian professional community.

CONTROVERSY

Horney was one of the first analysts to challenge basic Freudian assertions, such as the psychoanalytic account of female development. Based on her own understanding of herself as a woman, she took issue with the idea that women wish to be men because of an inferiority (i.e., they lack a penis), of their external genitals. According to classical Freudian theory women presumably then develop feelings of inadequacy. Horney stated that, while there are some women who desire to have a penis, their wish is not caused by a feeling of being castrated creatures. Rather, she asserted that the classical psychoanalytic perception of women's masculinity complex was a devaluation of women, the outcome of a male-dominated culture. Women, she advanced, have a tendency to define themselves in terms of men's needs and/or wishes. Horney went even further by postulating that men perceive women as having penis envy as a way of reducing their own inadequacy, their inability to creatively have a child.

Horney disputed Freudian psychoanalysis by challenging its biological, psychosexual premise. She saw behavior as a consequence of cultural distinctions and values, the outcome of a masculine-dominated society. She also criticized the prevailing psychoanalytic view that women are inherently more masochistic than men. She claimed that it was a cultural ideology that women feel weaker emotionally than men and are therefore more prone to self-destructive behavior. Probably Horney's experience of American culture in contrast to European culture gave her a clearer perspective that allowed her to reject the basic Freudian instinct theory in favor of cultural determinants.

Horney became disenchanted with the Freudian mandate that the patient's present behavior must inevitably be interpreted in terms of the past. Instead, she saw the value of concentrating on the present behavior in the context of character trends. Horney observed that all behavior was not sexual in origin nor was aggression necessarily bad; it could be mere assertion.

The preceding challenges to the Freudian dictum increasingly alienated and antagonized some influential members of the New York Psychanalytic institute. They pressured her to resign and she left, along with a number of sympathetic colleagues who appreciated free expression, exploration, and discussion of psychoanalytic contributions. They correctly recognized that psychoanalytic thought was a work in progress, not a completed body of knowledge.

Horney and the colleagues who left with her formed their own institute, the American Institute for Psychoanalysis and the Association for the Advancement of Psychoanalysis. At first, under the leadership of William Silverberg, there was collegial harmony and a free expression of diverse ideas. But when lay analyst Erich Fromm joined the institute, he was not accorded the same teaching of technique and supervisory rights as his medical colleagues. Relegated to a peripheral position, Fromm left the newly formed institute. A number of prominent analysts left with Fromm, among them Harry Stack Sullivan, Clara Thompson, and Janet Rioch. Horney was a prime mover in ousting Fromm. The two had been lovers and Horney may have been angry with him for ending their affair and for presumably driving a wedge presumably between her and her daughter, Marriane. Horney had referred her daughter to Fromm as her training analyst. Perhaps Horney feared that Fromm would take over the fledgling institute or perhaps she wished to preserve the medical aura of the institute for political reasons. It is possible Horney hoped for an affiliation with the New York Medical College. That hope never materialized.

Fromm's expulsion along with the departure of a number of talented, creative analysts may have retarded a more spirited advancement of psychoanalytic theory and technique within the institute. Nonetheless, under the leadership of Karen Horney and her remaining supporters, the institute thrived.

Horney's attitude toward nonmedical analysts is a puzzling one. When Horney left Europe and moved to London she sent her children to Melanie Klein, a lay analyst. She also respected and admired Fromm's psychoanalytic competence, since she sent her daughter to him for a training analysis. At that time, though, there were many psychoanalytic institutes which treated nonmedical students and applicants for psychoanalytic training as second-class citizens. Even Theodor Reik, a colleague of Freud, was refused full membership in the New York Psychoanalytic Institute on the grounds that he did not possess a medical degree.

Karen Horney continued to expand her institute in New York City until her death at 67 years of age. Horney died in her sleep from cancer on December 4, 1952. She left a remarkable professional legacy: the thriving Karen Horney Psychoanalytic Institute and Center at 329 East 92nd Street in New York City, which provides psychoanalytically oriented training programs for professionals in the mental health field under the auspices of the American Institute for Psychoanalysis (the institute and center also offers low-cost psychoanalytic psychotherapy); the *American Journal of Psychoanalysis*, a publication extending Horney's ideas and the contributions of other models of psychotherapy (e.g., existential). Her books, containing her ground-breaking psychoanalytic ideas, have gone through more than 19 printings, and a multitude of psychotherapists utilize her ideas in psychotherapy.

THE WRITING STYLE OF KAREN HORNEY

Karen Horney's writing is clear, well-organized, and engaging. Susan Quinn (1987, p. 266) notes that she had the ". . . knack for describing the experience of others in a way that is instantly recognizable to them, in a way that makes them feel, 'She's talking about me.'" Quinn (1988, p. 283) comments that, her lectures as well as her writings seemed to have a common impact of self-recognition on her audience and readers. They made comments such as "When I read her books, I saw myself," and "I felt as if she knew me and it helped me understand myself and others better."

Bernard J. Paris, a professor of English and a biographer of Horney, observes that her writing is not fashionably obscure in the vein of Lacan, Derrida, and post modernism.

> It is not full of mysterious, recondite terminology, as are the writings of Freud, Jung, and Lacan, and it does not have the aura of being secret knowledge possessed only by the master. It does not provide an elaborate analogical or mythological system that appears to explain the obscure or the ineffable. Much of it deals with what we can learn through self-observation rather than with highly inventive hypotheses about infantile and unconscious experience. Horney explores unconscious motives and conflicts, but she makes them readily accessible to conscious understanding. (Paris, 1994, pp. xx–xxi)

Dr. Cameron (1954, p. 29) a psychoanalytic psychiatrist cites

> . . . an important characteristic of Karen Horney's work; her essential directness and simplicity of approach to the problems on which she worked. One may attribute this to two things. First, she was not trapped, as so many others are and have been, in the theoretic superstructure of her teachers. And secondly, we must attribute Karen Horney's essential directness and simplicity of approach to the fact that she herself did not seem to require the successive development of theoretic structure which has been so much an impediment to the communication of others.

Dr. Cameron makes an observation concerning the development of analytic thinking which succinctly points up a failing in advancing analytic therapy, a failing Horney avoided. He (Cameron, 1954, p. 29) notes:

> It is quite tragic to see what a vast amount of labor has been spent in endlessly turning over and exchanging, with wearisome repetition, the thought forms of the original mind—thought forms from which the vitality has now departed as certainly as it has from an empty sea shell.

HORNEY'S BOOKS AND PAPERS

Between 1937 and 1950 Horney completed five books that contained her major ideas. Her first book was *The Neurotic Personality of Our Time*

(1937). This book heightened cultural awareness of mental illness. The second book, *New Ways in Psychoanalysis* (1939), critiqued Freud's premises and was responsible for her rejection by her New York analytic Freudian colleagues. Horney's third book, *Self-Analysis* (1942), details a case history of "Clare," illustrating the application of Horney's new model of psychoanalytic thinking. Both *Our Inner Conflicts* (1945) and *Neurosis and Human Growth* (1950a) advance Horney's views of basic anxiety, interpersonal and intrapsychic defenses. She also discusses the "pride system," self-hate, the search for glory, neurotic claims, tyrannical "shoulds," and the idealized self.

Feminine Psychology (1967) and *Final Lectures* (1987) were published after her death. *Feminine Psychology* disputed Freud's concept of penis envy, female masochism, and feminine development. *Final Lectures* (1987) contains transcripts of her concluding course dealing with psychoanalytic therapy.

Bernard J. Paris has performed an invaluable service for Horneyan clinicians by editing two books, *The Therapeutic Process* (1999), a collection of her clinical essays and lectures, and *The Unknown Karen Horney* (2000), a spectrum of her papers dealing with feminine psychology, relationships between the sexes, and psychoanalytic theory.

PLAN OF THE BOOK

To indroduce Horney's core ideas I shall rely chiefly on *Our Inner Conflicts* (1945) and *Neurosis and Human Growth* (1950a), as I believe they more than her other books best represent her theory and clinical thinking. I intend to offer clinical illustrations of her ideas as I encountered them in my practice. Whenever possible I shall try to keep the vignettes as brief as possible although there will be a few exceptions along the way. I shall also introduce the contributions of other psychoanalytic schools (e.g., Freudian, Kleinian) when they are relevant, although the preponderance of my interpretations and understanding will be along Horneyan lines. Given the complexity of human behavior it is foolish and downright unfair to a patient to slot that patient exclusively into one analytic model no matter how useful that model may or may not be. I shall always remember an American Psychological Association conference on various therapy models. Each school of therapy had a major representative and at the conclusion of their talk a question from the audience proposed the following: How would each of them allocate $50,000 given to their clinic for the hiring of therapists of a different persuasion from their own? Dr. David Wolpe, a conditioning behavior pioneer, said he would only hire therapists who adhered to his theory. Rudolph Ekstein, a Freudian, said that he had often wondered how a practitioner of another therapy model might succeed with patients he had failed to help. He would hire some therapists who had a different theoretical point of view than his own. I was quite impressed by his humility and appreciation of the complexity of behavior and the appropriate recognition that no one school of therapy possesses the total truth.

APPLYING HORNEY'S PRINCIPLES TODAY

The goals of this book are as follows:

1. To introduce, define, and illustrate through clinical vignettes the major tenets of Horney's theory and technique. Her treatment of self-hate is a good example. With regard to this formidable dynamic component within the self, Horney (1950a, p. 112) wrote, that it "makes visible a rift in the personality that started with the creation of an idealized self. It signifies that there is a war on." Horney also noted (p. 114) that "the *power and tenacity of self-hate* is astounding even for the analyst who is familiar with the way it operates." More than any other psychoanalyst Horney put into words the key role self-hate played in the character disorder's pathology. She stated: "Surveying self-hate and its ravaging force we cannot help but see it as a great tragedy, perhaps the greatest tragedy of the human mind" (p. 154).

2. To indicate how Horney's observation that there is a potential for growth existing in each individual fosters a powerful, optimistic attitude strengthening the cooperation in therapy between the therapist and the patient; It acts to restore the patient's expectation that constructive change can eventually occur.

3. To demonstrate the special suitability and effectiveness of Horney's ideas as they are applied to today's most frequent form of treatment, namely, one session per week psychotherapy. Horney, for example, emphasized attending to the here and now in the session and not becoming enmeshed in a Talmudic preoccupation with the patient's history. Horney alerted the mental health professional to vital global character trends such as effacement, expansiveness, and detachment and sensitized the therapist to the specific nuances and consequences of these global issues as they were played out interpersonally. One facet of detachment astutely noticed by her and excellently described (Horney, 1950a, p. 261) is the following:

> Even in the very first consultation he may, with the help of some pertinent questions, develop a picture of himself replete with a wealth of candid observation. But he will usually add that all this knowledge has not changed anything. No change because the detached individual is merely a dispassionate onlooker at himself.

4. To present criticisms of Horney's ideas and possible rebuttals to these judgments by Freudians, for example, that Horney neglects the patient's developmental history. However, Horney (1945, p. 218) found that "Even the most detailed recollection of his early experiences gives the patient little beyond a more lenient, more condoning attitude toward himself. It in no way makes his present conflicts any less disrupting."

2 The Basic Tenets of Karen Horney

Horney's major contribution to psychoanalytic therapy is her portrayal of the fine distinctions of character pathology. In this chapter I shall first define character disorder, present the basic tenets of Karen Horney's theory and technique, and contrast it with the main ideas of those analysts and psychologists who have also contributed to our understanding of character disorder, the most common dysfunction of our time.

Karen Horney was not the first ground-breaking psychoanalyst to observe and write about the significance of character disorder. There were other pioneering contemporaries of Horney who addressed the same pathology, such as Wilhelm Reich and Hellmuth Kaiser.

Almost 2 decades after Horney's death in 1952, Heinz Kohut (1971) presented his new ideas concerning the narcissistic personality, a character disorder. He postulated a grandiose self inherent in the narcissistic personality. It is distinguished by exhibitionism, expansiveness, and a sense of omnipotence. Horney, in her last book *Neurosis and Human Growth* (1950a), had succinctly captured the essence of the narcissistic character disorder when she wrote "More precisely: the person is his idealized self and seems to adore it. It gives him a seeming abundance of self confidence which appears enviable to all those chafing under self-doubts" (1950a, p. 194).

More recently psychologists such as Albert Ellis and M.E.P. Seligman have also added to our comprehension of character disorders.

THE INCREASE IN CHARACTER DISORDERS

The increase in the appearance of character disorder in the general pa-tient population since the 1970s and 1980s may in part be due to cul-tural changes. Lasch (1979) in a seminal book, *Culture of Narcissism*, details the main current thrust of our society: its emphasis on the su-perficial, material gratifications of the self and a burgeoning indiffer-ence for the concerns of others. An example of this now is the television series "The Apprentice" overseen by the seemingly "omnis-cient" CEO guru, Donald Trump, and other much more brutal, primi-tive narcissistic television "reality" shows. These entertainment contrivances eulogize successful, ruthless competition and narcissism in young adults.

DEFINITION OF CHARACTER DISORDER

In the *Neurotic Personality of Our Time*, Horney (1937, p. 31) first intro-duced the term "character neurosis," a deformation of the personality. Symptoms, she writes, in the clinical sense are absent although there is an underlying basic anxiety. Discussing treatment in *New Ways in Psychoanalysis*, Horney (1939, p. 283) uses a new term, "character struc-ture," and analyzes incompatible trends within the character structure. We see that Horney is more and more concentrating on character and its various subtle and overt manifestations.

Generally speaking, those with character disorders do not present distinct clinical symptoms, although they may express discontent with who they are and life in general. My clinical experience bears out Horney's observation that they do experience basic anxiety, depression, and mistrustful attitudes at some level.

The *Diagnostic Criteria from DSM-IV* (of the American Psychiatric Association, 1994, p. 275) defines the character disorder in ways that are strikingly similar to the character disorders described by Horney. The general definition emphasizes an enduring pattern of inner cognitive, af-fective, interpersonal, and impulse control that departs significantly from cultural expectations.

The Paranoid Personality, for example, that is listed under the heading of personality disorders in the DSM-IV is quite similar to Horney's expansive subtype, an arrogant-vindictive character disorder. The DSM-IV's Schizoid Personality resembles Horney's detached character disorder.

Further dwelling on the nature of character disorders, Horney in *Self-Analysis* (1942, p. 69) asserts that the primary basis of a "neurosis" is the neurotic character structure consisting of various character trends. If we piece together the various statements of Horney alluding to character we arrive at a comprehensive operational definition, namely, character disorder is the manifestation of a pattern of personality traits fueled by basic anxiety expressed through an individual's idiosyncratic self. The character disorder is made up of a tapestry of elements: the real self, alienation from self, "shoulds," idealized image, self-hate, claims, pride, anxiety, and conflicts.

BASIC TENETS OF KAREN HORNEY'S THEORY AND TECHNIQUE

1. Character disorder originates in part from cultural elements and distortions in interpersonal relationships. Specific cultural factors may determine an emphasis on certain character traits, such as aggressive competitiveness in relationships, work, love, or penis envy in women due to cultural chauvinism.

Horney (1937) offers an example of how the definition of what constitutes character pathology will change as a function of the passage of time. She states

> The conception of what is normal varies not only with the culture but also within the same culture, in the course of time. Today, for example, if a mature and independent women were to consider herself "a fallen woman," "unworthy of the love of a decent man" because she had had a sexual relationship, she would be suspected of a neurosis, at least in many circles of society. Some forty years ago, this attitude of guilt would have been considered normal (Horney, 1937, p. 15).

2. She rejects Freud's Instinct Theory because aggression and sexual pathology are caused by frustration of fundamental needs for love, safety, and security and by an increase in anxiety. Horney (1939, p. 71) concluded that

> The instinctual theory . . . leads to seeing final limitations in therapy where they do not exist. By regarding biological factors as the *ultimate causa movens* [author's italics], one is bound to come to rock bottom in therapy because as Freud points out, one cannot change what is determined by biology.

3. Character disorders always have basic anxiety as their cornerstone. The helplessness or basic anxiety of the child leaves him or her vulnerable with a conviction of being isolated and helpless in a possibly unkind world.

In Horney's first book, *The Neurotic Personality of Our Time* (1937), she declared that "anxiety is the dynamic center of neurosis and thus we shall have to deal with it all the time" (p. 41). Astute observations by Horney concerning the central role of anxiety continued, such as "by its very irrationality anxiety presents an implicit admonition that something within us is out of gear and therefore it is a challenge to overhaul something with ourselves" (Horney, p. 47).

She listed 3 fundamental "ways of escaping anxiety; rationalize it; deny it; avoid thoughts, feelings, impulses and situations which might arouse it" (Horney, 1937, pp. 47–48). Horney went on to state "In fact, *hostile impulses of various kinds are the main source from which neurotic anxiety springs* [italics added]." She suggested an optimal attitude of the therapist to dealing with anxiety:

> whenever I find anxiety or indications of it, the questions that come to my mind are, what sensitive spot has been hurt and has consequently provoked hostility, and what accounts for the neccessity of repression? My experience is that a search in these directions often leads to a satisfactory understanding of anxiety (Horney, p. 77).

4. Mankind has the ability as well as the desire to evolve into a reasonable human being. An individual can change and go on changing as long as he lives. Inherent in man is a desire to fulfill his given potentialities, a drive for self-realization.

The Horneyan American Institute For Psychoanalysis' catalogue of course content begins with the following quote from Horney's book *Neurosis and Human Growth*, which is in the first paragraph of this work. It epitomizes her optimistic attitude toward the patient's prospect of positive change and the basis for her theory and psychotherapy technique.

> You need not, and in fact cannot teach an acorn to grow into an oak tree, but when given a chance, its intrinsic potentialities will develop. Similarly, the human individual, given a chance tends to develop his particular human potentialities (Horney, 1950a, p. 17).

5. There is a need to value oneself and to be valued. Poor self-esteem is a consequence of either under- or over-valuation of the self. This leads to a specific idealized image by way of compensation. Horney points out that sometimes an over-evaluation of the self in the form of idealizing fantasies can play a positive role in maintaining emotional stability. Horney (1939, p. 93) writes "My personal impression is that the illusions do far more than give secret substitute satisfactions. I often wonder whether they do not save the individual from being crushed entirely and thus whether they are not literally life-saving."

6. Horney defined conflict broadly, seeing it as either a juxtaposition between the real self versus the idealized image, the real self versus the pride system, or the destructive forces versus the constructive urges.

7. The treatment of the present in therapy is immeasurably more effective than the focus on the past. This tenet is similar to the focus on the present by cognitive therapists.

In a sense Horney's model is analogous to looking at a building as if it was a patient. General features of the building are first noticed, such as size, color, place, style, and shadows cast affecting other neighboring buildings. The sizes of the rooms, nature of their layout, and inner building materials are necessarily slighted momentarily. This perspective may be all that is needed for successful psychotherapy. I supply an abundance of clinical material that supports Horney's model. However, the therapist can borrow other useful concepts from different analytic schools to add detail and dynamics neglected by Horney's theory. For example, she omits the treatment of identifications, that is, whom the patient internalized (i.e., a representation of a person psychically swallowed). A knowledge of the clash of identifications within the self can prove vital to effective therapy. The Kleinian exposition (Solomon, 1995) of projective identification and introjection may help explain many vexing transference and counter-transference issues.

OTHER CONTRIBUTORS TO THE UNDERSTANDING OF CHARACTER DISORDER

Horney's contemporary, Wilhelm Reich (1933), in his pioneering work *Character Analysis* perceived character as a series of resistances one on top of another. According to him, the patient's ego defends against id impulses. He recognized that free association does not work with character disorders, nor does making the unconscious conscious. He suggested that resistances be interpreted first. How the patient resists therapy represents to Reich, character, a protective "armor." Horney would agree with Reich that resistances need to be attended to. However, she would add an additional important element to bringing a resistance to the patient's awareness, that his "awareness of consequences is the most powerful curative factor in analysis in that only by changing certain things within himself can he ever attain freedom" (Horney, 1945, p. 177).

Richard F. Sterba (1953) criticized Reich for equating resistance with character. He also disputed Reich's conclusion that the initial transference is a form of resistance and should be dealt with as such. According to Sterba, however, a positive transference may be genuine and made up of ambivalent impulses including forerunners of love. Sterba objects to Reich's concept of a neat layer of resistance. He concluded that our psychic apparatus is not "neatly" layed out but is the product of faults much like geological disruptions. Character, for Sterba, goes beyond the activity of resistance but is the total expression of the id, ego, and superego. Anna Freud's (1946) definition of character is more to Sterba's liking. She perceived character as a cluster of ongoing attitudes of the individual's ego to solve perpetual inner conflicts. She emphasized the defensive aspect of the patient's ego.

Hellmuth Kaiser (1955) conceptualizes character resistance in terms of self-esteem. The more a patient displays inappropriate behavior, the more we perceive character resistance. Character resistance is impersonal, a particular style in nature, such as the "defiant character."

Akin to Horney's idea of claim, Kaiser states that for the "defiant character" merely having the claim of moral superiority brings gratification and/or a sense of importance.

Kaiser advocates consistent pursuit of resistance analysis. The character disorder has a "fortress" of resistances and the therapist has to help the patient become aware of the what and how this "fortress" is manifested. It seems to me that Reich again affirms Horney's emphasis on addressing the present what and how of "blockages" within a firm therapeutic alliance. The therapeutic alliance for Kaiser is based on elements of tender attachment transference to the therapist. Like Horney, Kaiser stresses dealing with immediacy, that is the what and how that is occurring in the present.

More recently Paul (1989, pp. 125–126), a Horneyan psychoanalyst, compared and contrasted Horney and Kohut (1971, 1977). Both saw neurosis originating from the anxiety of parent-child issues. Kohut, however, perceived fixation and regression, Freudian concepts, as predominantly genetic features of neurosis.

Both Kohut and Horney were convinced that each person had potentially within him or herself a growth-oriented self, and that this self could be liberated. Horney's real self was made up of intrinsic healthy forces, whereas Kohut's nuclear self was a bipolar structure (i.e., a self made up of two poles, one being ambitions, the other ideals) linked to specific developmental lines and well-defined transference advances. Horney explains character structure and its pathology as a result of a conflict between injured pride or frustrated claims and the idealized image. Kohut, by contrast, conceptualizes character disorder as a narcissistic regression and/or fixation.

Horney advises attention in treatment to all the patient's obstructive forces. Kohut (1971), adhering to the libido theory, writes about aiding the patient to gradually withdraw narcissistic libido from the narcissisitically invested archaic object ("object" is the classical analytic term for person).

Karen Horney has also influenced two of today's most popular psychologists, Albert Ellis and Martin Seligman.

Albert Ellis (1963), a combination of behavior and cognitive therapist, like Horney emphasizes the present. He postulates that inherent in each individual there is a self-actualizing potentiality akin to Horney's real self. He acknowledges that culture plays an important role transmitted through one's parents. He asserts that there is also an inherent self-destructive drive. By contrast, Horney under the rubric of self-hate would see self-destructiveness as inevitably emerging out of childhood anxieties and insecurities.

There are major fundamental differences between Horney and Ellis, including their approach to resistances. Ellis advocates a blunt, aggressive assault on the patient's resistances. To portray what he considers the correct therapeutic posture to resistances, he employs colorful, aggressive language, such as "keep hacking away at it," "blasting away," the use of explentitives. If Horney were to engage in a dialogue with Ellis I surmise that she would inform him that the patient's knowledge of his blockages may be more important than what he is defending against. And in all humility I would say that sometimes the patient's resistances are more a function of the therapist's lack of empathy or countertransference issues. Ellis does recognize that the character disorder's "must haves" and "shoulds" need to be delineated and ultimately confronted, as Horney noted. However, Horney would probably think that encouraging the therapist to verbally assault a resistant patient to remove a resistance is a slippery slope. It may give permission to latent sadistic, punitive impulses residing in the therapist or gratify the masochistic patient.

Psychologist Martin Seligman (1991) in his book *Learned Optimism* does not mention Horney's (1945) treatment of hopelessness in *Our Inner Conflicts*, even though he is most concerned with effective treatment of depression Seligman, more specifically, saw "learned helplessness" as its basis. Central to the concept of learned helplessness is despair. Horney also perceived undue dependency on others as predisposing an individual to depression and despair. She found that any failure experienced by some character disorders was perceived as a magnified inadequacy, pessimism, and unrealistic, idealized goals. In Horney's model the idealized image plays a central role forcing the character disorder to strive for perfection; the end result is usually depression.

Seligman also sees learned helplessness, a concomitant of depression, in the service of a pessimistic style. He celebrates the virtue of optimism, especially as an antidote to depression. Basically Seligman found that the depressive individual feels he has no control over his future. But the lack of control, as Horney (1945) observes, is the character disorder's alienation from his real self and his giving up on his own capacity to change his life for the better. He has through dependency shifted responsibility for change, and his morbid dependency becomes the chief cause of despair.

We will further experience through clinical vignettes the important implications of the enumerated tenets underlying Horney's theory and technique. They will be demonstrated in the following chapters as they come to light.

3 Horneyan Theory and Clinical Insights

The purpose of this chapter is to present some aspects of Horney's basic theoretical model and illustrations of her impressive clinical insights. My presentation will be augmented by relevant clinical vignettes. I may at times return to the same patient material to highlight a point that was not previously and extensively discussed.

I will begin with a vital element of therapy, despair, that must be overcome in any course of therapy if treatment will be ultimately successful.

HOPELESSNESS

Horney (1945) devotes an entire chapter to hopelessness in her book *Our Inner Conflicts*. Her attention to this vital issue and how she delineates its vicissitudes is to my mind a wonderful example of her keen, insightful attunement to the subtleties of behavior.

She begins by pointing out the neurotic's vulnerability caused by undue dependency on others and entangling conflicts (e.g., wishes and contradictory objections to those wishes).

Any failure or mishap is magnified and perceived as evidence of inadequacy. The neurotic becomes involved in a script characterized by "What ifs." Thus he keeps saying to himself "What if I had married someone else, had a better job, a different career, loving parents?" These scripts

21

generate hopelessness because the character disorder repeatedly convinces him that any material or external change will cause him to feel so much better about himself. Of course, the plastic surgery, the move to another house, the new marriage replacing the previous marriage, does not work, for the "should," prides, and solutions just follow him to a new situation (Horney, 1945, p. 180).

The following vignette describes a patient's clinging to a vain hope and imagining that gratification of that externally based hope will bring her happiness.

Linda imagined that Bill, a man she had loved in the past and who had not committed to her, would now make a better husband than her present husband. The former lover would allow her to overcome her conviction that she could not alter her life in a positive way. If somehow he would divorce his wife and return to her, life would be complete. Many years had passed and Linda had no inkling at all of her former lover's state of mind, but he was now seen as the antidote to her hopelessness. If he came back into her life, Linda then would not have to assume any responsibility for changing her life. Her former lover's continued absence from her life could justify her persistent despair.

The next vignette focuses on the effects of maternal negative feedback and the formation of hopelessness.

When she was a child Tammy was told by her mother that she was "cheap goods" or inadequate. Therefore, she felt that anything that went wrong in her life was caused by her inherently bad make-up. Her mother's repeated comments about Tammy's supposed inherited inadequacy carried special weight since in Tammy's mind her mother was so good at spotting defects. How then could she ever change her life for the better given her basic limitations? The future could only be viewed by her with despair.

There are clues to a patient's potential to dive into hopelessness and Horney suggests some possible signs: A history of periods of deep despair set off by what appear to be inconsequential occurrences, a preoccupation with death, a refusal to take anything seriously, and regressing in therapy after a progressive, healthy, forward movement. Horney calls this type of regression or resurgence of symptoms the "Negative Therapeutic Reaction."

Horney correlated a wish to foresee the future with underlying hopelessness. Since the future is expected to be bad the gift of fortune telling would avoid any future fatality. Being able to step around forthcoming mishaps offers supreme control over any bad consequences and helps maintain an optimistic, hopeful attitude.

Hopelessness, according to Horney, is associated with depression, a feeling of impending doom, resignation, and life as a tragedy. The patient caught in the grip of despair feels paralyzed and unable to take even the slightest risk to improve his lot. Repeated failures to change positively evoke and reinforce chronic discouragement.

Horney is convinced that the neurotic's idealized image plays a large role in fostering hopelessness. Horney (1945, p. 184) notes that hopelessness occurs when the patient recognizes that he can not be the perfect person he so longs to be. Instead he is just another imperfect mortal among other imperfect mortals. This awareness brings him depression and self-hate.

Hopelessness causes the patient to become alienated from his real self. No one notices that there is a psychic death taking place, covered over by a seemingly decent adaptation to life. Horney rightly emphasizes that the therapist himself must not succumb to hopelessness. There has to be a belief that the patient can unleash his potentialities. I am reminded by Horney's underscoring of potentiality of Michelangelo's answer to the question "How do you approach a stone to create such a magnificent sculpture?" He is reported to have said, "The sculpture is already there in the stone. I merely free it."

Horney advises that the patient's hopelessness must be taken seriously but that the therapist has to become aware and make clear to the patient that his plight is not unchangeable. As long as he persists in viewing his situation as hopeless, no change will take place. A patient once said to me, "I feel that I am in a tunnel and I don't know if I will ever get out. Will I?" I responded with "It depends on what attitude you have as you go into the tunnel."

The psychoanalyst Donald Winnicott, who was not an adherent to Horney's theory, echoes her optimism when he suggests an interesting and novel therapeutic approach to severe despair. He (Winnicott, 1974, pp. 103–107) advises that the therapist invite the patient to consider and possibly recall that in the past he had once gone through a similar period of despair and successfully extricated himself from that travail, although the patient has probably repressed this triumph. If he had accomplished it once in the past he could extricate himself from hopelessness again.

The therapist must strenuously call upon his own inner sustainment so that he or she can hold on to the anchor of hope. As I (Solomon, 1992, p. 136) stated in a past paper

> In the face of hopelessness the analyst (substitute therapist) must re-connect with those stressful personal moments, where he or she once felt despair, survived, and even prospered. The analyst must be immersed in the transience of all pain and pleasure, share the patient's despair, yet know too that all affect is mortal. Also, an analyst must take comfort in the dialect of hope. Without its reality, there could be no negation called despair. Also a therapist is, by nature, the stubborn personification of potential.

We shall repeatedly see that an admirable, inspiring premise of Horney is her heartfelt conviction and observation that patients have within them a constructive energy that, when tapped, urges them toward productive, inner freedom from the shackles of neurosis.

ENVY AND HOPELESSNESS

Horney in her first book *The Neurotic Personality of Our Time* (1937) mentioned the vital role of envy as it maintained hopelessness. She stated "The neurotic, whether or not he feels it consciously, is not only a very unhappy person indeed, but he does not see any chance of escaping his misery" (Horney, 1937, p. 227). Horney described the neurotic as if "being hopelessly caught in a net." What the therapist or other outside observers may see as "vicious circles really are developed out of attempts to get reassurance," to escape hopelessness. According to Horney (1939, p. 228),

> gradually developing hopelessness is the basis from which envy is constantly generated. It is not so much an envy of something special, but

what Nietzsche has described as *Lebensneid*, a very general envy of everyone who feels more secure, more poised, more happy, more straightforward, more self-confident.

Although Horney does not take this next logical step, it would seem to me that a therapist, who hopefully is more self-confident and secure than the patient, would ultimately be envied by the patient.

BLAME

In any case, whether the character disorder is or is not aware of his hopelessness, he will attempt to deal with it. Horney (1937, pp. 228–229) noted that

> He does not see it—as the analytical observer does—as the outcome of an inexorable process. Instead he sees it caused by others or by himself. My clinical experience has been that the character disorder will usually blame others for his despair.

Horney (1937, p. 229) observed "When he puts the blame on others an accusatory attitude results, which may be directed toward fate in general, toward circumstances or toward special persons: parents, teachers, husband, physician."

Blaming others for their hopelessness absolves the character disorder and shifts the responsibility for change away from themselves. Horney (1939, p. 229) remarks "It is as if the neurotic thought along these lines: 'Since you are all responsible for my suffering, it is your duty to help me, and I have a right to expect it from you.'" A patient in the grip of this type of thinking may then accuse the therapist of incompetence and a lack of empathic understanding. Of course, there is always the possibility that the therapist may not be in touch with the vital elements in the patient's character deformation. Horney (p. 229) points out with regard to the patient:

> there are also neurotic elements in his accusations: they often take the place of constructive efforts toward positive goals and usually they are blind and indiscriminate. They may be directed, for example, toward

persons who want to help him and at the same time he may be entirely incapable of feeling and expressing accusations against those persons who really injure him.

Horney (1939, p. 264) suggests that "Because of his compulsory unobtrusiveness and dependency, with all their implications, molehills often appear to him as mountains, particularly when he is supposed to do something for himself, or when he is faced with responsibilities or risks."

The patient Wendy voiced despair at ever meeting a suitable man. When I questioned her as to what she was doing to meet men, she presented a list of possible barriers, cutting off any productive efforts of her own. Men became in her eyes "giant ogres" who would reject her. Meeting a man for her was akin to moving a mountain—an illustration of Horney's (1939) clinical observation that character disorders exaggerate in their imagination the obstacles to change.

The following is a vignette illustrating the many facets of hopelessness and how Horney's insights in general lead to greater understanding of the patient's dynamics.

When Milton entered treatment he was depressed, lonely, and vindictively angry at both his wife and daughter. At 45 years of age he felt life was empty and he could look forward only to more despair. As he sat alone drinking, he brooded over his daughter's lack of love for him and his wife's selfishness. It appeared to him that his wife merely kept him as an "escort," and his daughter considered him only as just another source of income. His despair was fueled by his penchant for blaming others, as Horney (1939, p. 228) observed.

Milton had become so embittered that his face was lined deeply with a perpetual scowl. He himself noted that people were constantly asking him if he was depressed or angry when he believed that he felt none of these feelings at the time. He wondered why the tiny group of his friends would flare up at him after what appeared to him to be a rather innocuous remark. Horney (1945, p. 205) would say "Since his righteousness prevents him from seeing his share in any difficulty that arises he must feel that he is the one who is abused and victimized; since he cannot see that the source of all his despair lies within himself he must hold others responsible for it."

Everyone, it seemed to him, frequently misunderstood his good intentions and appeared to attribute arrogant, vindictive motives to him. Milton was not aware of how hopelessness caused a pervasive character trend of vindictiveness. Horney (1937, p. 228) points out that it is very difficult for the despairing individual to have any sympathy for those he feels have spoiled his life and who in addition are in a superior emotional place to himself. I interpreted that Milton was more provocative out of envy towards people he perceived as more successful or more satisfied with their lives than he was.

At one point in therapy, Milton, more aware of his detachment, dreamed the following:

"I was sitting on a chair in a hospital room (I may have been a patient myself). On one side of me was a woman who had had a stroke. She was a patient in my wife's room. In reality her case was hopeless but in the dream she was improved. The other woman I noticed after a while was losing blood, which was flowing from a cut on her wrist."

To "losing blood" he associated losing what appeared to be a description of his idealized image, a flimsy pretense of great adequacy that was slowly fading away. We, his wife, daughter, and myself, were all perceived by him transferentially as demanding persecutors, more successful and more adequate than himself, lying in the wings. He was a perpetual, vulnerable, and envious victim. His situation would remain hopeless, he considered, as long as we (therapist, wife, daughter, friends, boss) might demand enviously all the success he obtained through his idealized image, pride, claims and "shoulds." According to Milton's psychological bookkeeping any advance made by him in therapy was just so much more of his success that I would forcefully extract from him.

My "raping" him in effect of his added growth fits in with Horney's (1936, p. 65) view of the negative therapeutic reaction (NTR). NTR refers to the impairment of a patient's condition after he has just made progress. Horney observed that

> the patients felt endangered in their own position and react with rage when the analyst does have a better grasp of the situation than they themselves. They must express their hostility and their sense of defeat by defeating the analyst. (p. 64)

I interpreted that Milton felt humiliated and competitively "weaker" than me in accordance with Horney's thinking on the connection between the patient's envy, NTR, and anger toward the therapist. My shared insights into Milton's character structure caused him to feel anger and humiliation; I, in his eyes, knew more about him than he did and this made him anxious. I emphasized that I was not triumphing over him with my understanding and, as Horney puts it, not making him *"a possible feather in the analyst's cap"* (1936, p. 64).

I will discuss dreams in more detail from the Horneyan perspective in a succeeding chapter but Horney's basic premise is illustrated in Milton's dreams. She wrote (1950a, p. 330) *"We know that in dreams our unconscious imagination can create solutions for an inner conflict that is disquieting us for the time being."* In the dream of Milton there is a conflict between the healthy self and the vindictive self (i.e., containing his helplessness and hopelessness). The constructive solution was to care for his wife in his dream; to give to her and improve her well-being. I told him that this was a healthy part of his self that truly cared for her.

In the dream Milton saw himself as a paralyzed woman, a defeated self. He could not budge from what he considered an intolerable, helpless, and hopeless position. All his dreams of glory were not being met. He had not become a doctor, a career goal he had longed to attain, nor had he made a great deal of money. Concurrently his wife, upon whom he depended more than he realized, was in reality in the hospital. The healthy part of his self wished her well. He needed her (in his dream "She was improved"), but another part of him, a vindictive aspect, desired her death. His wife, he believed, did not respect him. He offered the proof that she did not respect him with the following observations: When he stated his opinion among a group of their friends, for example, she would always ask for another viewpoint as if she could not accept the possibility that his opinion could be correct. She also did not seem to notice slights directed against him by her friends. If she did, when he brought it to her attention, she would minimize the offense or she would say he was overreacting.

However, beneath Milton's despair and hostility connected to the self-hating aspect of his self and typical of a character disorder, there still lurked a strong, sadistic, vindictive trend. He was unconsciously clinging to hopelessness as a consequence of not getting excessive regard from others as a victim. He was consciously adamant that he was being stressed by his unfeeling wife, his exploiting daughter, and the ineffectual therapist.

Horney (1945, pp. 110–111) would probably hypothesize that Milton

> is dependent upon endless affirmation from others in the form of approval and admiration, flattery—none of which, however, can give him any more than temporary reassurances. He may unconsciously hate everyone who is overbearing or, better than he is any way—more assertive, more evenly balanced, better informed—threatening to undermine his own notions of himself. The more desperately he clings to the belief that he is his idealized image, the more violent the hatred.

His self-hatred increases because his narcissism, bolstering his idealized image, is being undermined by his perception of individuals considered more "superior" in certain ways than himself. His own conscious experience was that of a despairing, circumspect, vigilant, self-effacing, sensitive, considerate husband and father (i.e., his idealized self). In sum, his capacity to externalize (i.e., projection onto others of his own behavior, seeing other as treating him unfairly while in reality he provoked them) was working fast and furiously. Therefore, the following dream, revealing a grotesque malignity within him, really startled him:

> *"I dreamed that I electrocuted the porter, a tall black man. I applied electrodes by hand while he was on a hospital stretcher. He would not utter a sound. I applied the electrodes several times and watched the pallor set in. I was vaguely aware that there was someone alongside me."*

The patient, to his chagrin (i.e., the consequences of a sensitive, considerate idealized image vs. sadistic, torturing idealized image), was now confronted in the dream with his obvious sadism where he was at the same time, the gleeful, dispassionate torturer, the idealized image (i.e., the torturer), and the tortured (i.e., the black man, his poor, victimized self). His associations confirmed this divided role. He remembered that as an adolescent he felt trapped and despairing when his uncles had exploited him, employing him in their factory to carry heavy burdens and paying him very little. He was indeed the "porter" to them, represented by the "porter" in the dream. He associated that he was also "shocking" himself as a way of mitigating his hopelessness, a means also of erasing his emotional numbness. Instead of "emotional numbness," Horney (1945, p. 185) would employ as a description "psychic death." In another place, Horney (p. 207) refers to the despairing, hopeless character disorder as "so dead that he needs these sharp stimuli to feel alive." The patient recalled that during his latency years, he would enjoy picking wings off insects, a sadistic urge he had sublimated through biology laboratory work. He also "picked" at people in the same manner as he handled the insects, to provoke them and see how much they could take. As Horney (p. 206) asserts: "In degrading others he not only allays his intolerable self-contempt but at the same time gives himself a feeling of superiority." And "Last but not least, his sadistic dealings with others provide him with a feeling of strength and pride which reinforce his unconscious feeling of omnipotence" (Horney, p. 207). In addition, he wanted to see how much immunity he possessed against their possible retaliations. He tested out the strength of his vulnerability as a victim, provoked them and triumphed over them as his defeated persecutors. I was perceived by him transferentially as another persecutor, the "someone" in the dream vaguely alongside him. I told him that he seemed to be a suffering human being who was filled with the conviction that he could not change his life for the better. However, he and I together could work at conquering his problem as a mere puzzle, able to be solved as he had successfully dealt with challenges in the past. In saying this I was echoing Horney (p. 216), who wrote the following about the patient who feels hopeless: He was "a desperate individual who seeks restitution for a life that has defeated him," and "his hopelessness does not spring from a factually hopeless situation but constitutes a problem to be understood and eventually solved" (Horney, p. 226).

Shortly before therapy ended, the patient brought in the following dream, an excellent example of Horney's (1939, p. 32) assertion that "In neurosis the most important function of dreams is the attempt to find either reassurance for an anxiety or compromise solutions for conflicts insoluble in real life." The dream was stimulated by a session in which he voiced increasing responsibility for his hopelessness and recognized that he was unfairly blaming others for the barrenness of his life.

"I was on an observation deck. My camera lens was scratched. A photo serviceman gave me a cold patch for the lens. I put the lens in a potted tree to fix the camera. The 'camera tree' would grow to fix the lens. I remember the roots of the tree were a vivid yellow, orange, and red."

This dream confirms the useful aspects of dreams. As Horney (1950a, pp. 349–350) indicates,

> From dreams with constructive elements the patient can catch a glimpse even in the initial phase of analysis, of a world operating within him which is peculiarly his own and which is more true to his feelings than the world of presses his illusions. There are dreams in which the patient expresses in symbolic form the sympathy he feels for himself because of what he is doing to himself. There are dreams which reveal a deep well of sadness, of nostalgia, of longing; dreams in which he is struggling to come alive; dreams in which he realizes that he is imprisoned and wants to get out; dreams in which he tenderly cultivates a growing plant or in which he discovers a room in his house of which he did not know before.

Getting back to the patient's dream, he associated to "observation deck" being up high, watching people, a good view, exposing himself to the world and home. The "scratched lens," we concluded from his associations, was himself, his real self impaired by life and his own self-hating, self-delusional actions. I was the "photo service man," he acknowledged, who had helped him to grow. Like the "camera tree" in his dream, he could now experience life as a tapestry of diverse, warm feelings such as "a vivid yellow, orange, and red" as in his dream. He did not see life as if it were predominantly a mosaic of drab grays and blacks. He recognized that his claims had been reinforcing overly critical, punitive attitudes (shoulds) that were alienating his family and friends. Milton could accept responsibility for perpetuating his hopelessness. He could now also perceive the virtues of his wife and daughter and not be driven so compulsively to be a vindictive judge of others. Finally, with the lifting of his depression, he could involve himself in outside interests, such as photography, which utilized his excellent, critical intelligence and passionate enthusiasm. More importantly, the patient was firmly convinced that he truly "owned" his real self, his goodness, and since he no longer perceived others transferentially as persecutors they could not take any success he obtained away from him.

THE IDEALIZED IMAGE

According to Horney, the neurotic constructs a fanciful image of what he feels he can or ought to be. This illusory image that is exalted renders the character disorder defenseless and conceited. Since his image is deceptive, a pressing search for outside affirmation is launched.

Largely unconscious the idealized image requires extraordinary strivings which are often mistaken for laudable, high standards. The character disorder becomes increasingly more convinced that he is special and outstanding. The real self is looked down upon and scorned. He drives himself to become his idealized self with a multitude of "shoulds," such as, to be more perfect, more intelligent. Since sensible limitations are ignored or berated, genuine growth is prevented.

The idealized self causes emotional damage by weakening self-confidence and reducing self-determination. Instead of the patient's real self making decisions, the idealized image is in the driver's seat. Further undesirable consequences follow: feelings of vindictive triumph, or hypersensitivity to being humiliated and the establishment of rigidity. In her last book, *Neurosis and Human Growth* (1950a), Horney was convinced that the idealized image of the character disorder was a potent engine of destruction. She stated

> I now saw gradually that the neurotic's idealized image did not merely constitute a false belief in his value and significance; it was rather like the creation of a Frankenstein monster which in time usurped his best energies, usurped his drive to grow, to realize his given potentialities. And this meant that he was no longer interested in realistically tackling or outgrowing his difficulties, and in fulfilling his potentials, but was bent on actualizing his idealized self. It entails not only the compulsive drive for worldly glory through success, power, and triumph but also the tyrannical inner system by which he tries to mold himself into

a godlike being; it entails neurotic claims and the development of neurotic pride. (Horney, p. 368)

The following vignette depicts an idealized image of a patient who is rigidly driven to lecture relentlessly to all and sundry to obtain admiration and attention.

Olivia's idealized image was that of an instructor in all the correct ways of living a supremely caring, competent, giving existence. Toward that end she was ever ready to dispense useful facts and what she considered her own personal dramatic and didactic experiences in a flat, droning voice.

Since Olivia was a little girl she had always wanted to be a teacher. She relished her childhood experiences when a teacher chose her to read to the class. She would imagine then that she was really the teacher and her classmates were both admiring and envious of her special status. She fulfilled her fantasy and ultimately did become a teacher, but now that she was retired she was feeling depressed and aimlessly drifting. She had no close friends and her marriage was filled with tension and anger. She could not fathom why her husband lashed out at her periodically and why any friendship she formed melted quickly away.

In session after session Olivia droned on and on, lecturing me on various topics ranging from the climate in Venezuela to direction to a nearby restaurant serving a particularly good roast beef. I began to feel some sympathy for her husband and her former friends as I discovered firsthand her part in getting others to become irritated with her and ultimately rejecting.

Olivia never left the lecturer's podium. She did not listen and sounded as if she knew more about any subject than anyone else, especially more than her husband. In my mind's eye, I could picture her husband gritting his teeth and rolling his eyes as he stifled increasing exasperation. The dam would break eventually and he would erupt into violent rages to Olivia's amazement.

I began my first intervention concerning Olivia's idealized image by describing how her compulsive need to be liked and admired for being a reliable dispenser of facts and solutions might not always be welcomed. I suggested that she think about the possible connection between her husband's rageful outburst, the disappearance of her friends due to her rigid idealized image of teacher, and her automatic perception of her friends as a grateful audience of appreciative students. I tried to help her see that she torpedoed any possibility of a spontaneous interchange of respectful feelings and ideas by forcing the other into the role of an angry, straight-jacketed student. "Of course," I said, "they would be angry and certainly not grateful since they had not signed up to take a course with you as their teacher."

My intervention was met by a barrage of rationalizations or, as Horney would put it, "blockages." Olivia defended her idealized image by attacking her husband's competence regarding decision making. She has rationalized her need to make all his choices for him. She said that he easily becomes rattled, feels insecure, and if she knows a better way why should she withhold this knowledge. She continued "If I was on the receiving end of useful information I would be grateful." I countered with two points addressing her entitlement to be arrogant and narcissistic. "Not everyone is like you." And "They did not ask you to educate them. It's demeaning. Consider the consequences: that is your husband's angry response and that of those individuals who drop you as a friend."

Olivia retorted with "I mean well." I answered in a way calculated to reduce a possible burgeoning of her self-hate with "Yes, you do and basically your real self is that of a caring person, but I'm merely inviting you to pause and take a longer look at how you express your caring and need for approval and what follows afterward."

The idealized image is created to wipe out conflicts and the acknowledgement of shortcomings. Were they to emerge they would evoke too much anxiety. The idealized image is like a precious suit of armor which the character disorder will fight "tooth and nail" to preserve.

The next vignette demonstrates the tenacity with which a patient will cling to an idealized image. The vignette also illustrates the difference between healthy ideals or goals and the unconstructive urges of the idealized image. Horney (1945, p. 98) states "In contrast to authentic ideals, the idealized image has a static quality, It is not a goal toward whose attainment he strives but a fixed idea which he worships."

The patient, Ida, was depressed and tearful over the latest frustrating encounter with her son. In his usual manner he had treated her shabbily and insensitively. She wanted to arrive at a state of mind where she would no longer be hurt by him. What prevented her from reaching this goal was her idealized image of herself as a person who could successfully reach anybody through her persistent, affectionate overtures.

Failing to reach her son, she fell into a deep pool of self-hate and saw her life as not worth living. Despite being loved by her three daughters, her son's callous treatment of her caused her to wallow and weep in self-pity. During the last phase of therapy, when she was able to challenge the unreality of her pursuit of a glorious reconciliation with her son, an unswerving requirement of her idealized image, she could finally enjoy the remaining years of her life and let in the good that her loving daughters were offering her.

The following vignette illustrates the patient's dawning awareness of the existence of a submerged idealized image responsible for underlying feelings of superiority. Note that the consequences of the idealized image are also shown in this vignette. Horney (1945, p. 109) declares about the character disorder that

> As long as his image remains real to him and intact, he can feel significant, superior and harmonious, in spite of the illusory nature of those feelings. He can consider himself entitled to raise all kinds of demands and claims on the basis of his assumed superiority. But if he allows it to be undermined he is immediately threatened with the prospect of facing all his weaknesses, with no title to special claims, a comparatively insignificant figure or even in his own eyes—a contemptible one.

Shortly after a dear friend had died, Fran shared with me that she was filled with ambivalent feelings regarding her deceased friend. While Fran missed her friend, she also recalled how this same friend thought she was indispensable to Fran. She believed that Fran, for example, could not find her way about town without her help. This deprecating attitude festered in the patient, since she never dared to confront her friend with her failure to give her the proper respect due to an equal, a competent adult.

However, as treatment proceeded Fran exposed a submerged idealized image of omniscience. She did feel superior to most people, she believed, because of her high intelligence. She found that she had a powerful need to feel exceptional. She saw this feature in her relationship to her colleagues. Any sign that a co-worker knew more than she did threw her into a depression. Her recognition of the link between the occurrence of depression and the need to fulfill the mandate of her idealized image, that is the maintenance of supremacy, led her to the nature of her idealized image (i.e., her chronic self-hate and defensive, competitive perfectionism). Fran saw more clearly how her overdemandingness, self-hate, and pride in her desire for excellence cramped her performance at work and limited her ability to have a decent relationship with others. She became more aware of how her idealized image caused her feeling entitled to be overcritical of others and of herself.

The following vignette presents a relationship between the idealized image embodying stifled, murderous rage and a physical symptom, migraine headaches. In this connection Horney (1937, p. 57) mentioned the effects of anxiety on our physical well-being. In *The Neurotic Personality of Our Time* she states that "anxiety produces a feeling of strain, fatigue or exhaustion." Rubins, a biographer of Horney, writes (1978, p. 196) that

> Certainly she accepted that many somatic symptoms, including muscle tension, were caused by conflict, even as Groddeck and Simmel (i.e., colleagues of Horney in the very early years of her psychoanalytic career in Europe) had insisted. In fact during her analytic work she would often send the patient to a physiotherapist for concurrent exercise, dance therapy, relaxation work or massage . . . therapy.

Discussing externalization of rage, Horney (1945, p. 121) observed that

> Rage against the self, when not expressed as such, apparently creates physical tensions of considerable severity, which many appear as intestinal maladies, headaches, fatigue, and so on. It is illuminating to see how all these symptoms disappear with the speed of lightening as soon as the rage is consequently felt.

When Larry related to his wife, he was soft spoken and meek. Most of his friends, wife, and family saw him as a "wimp" or passive. Larry was also afflicted with terrible migraines so severe that he had to keep a cot in his office when they occurred. Migraines were the chief basis for his entering treatment.

At one point Larry revealed that he had had a repetitive dream ever since he was an adolescent. For weeks at a time he dreamt each night that he was on a rooftop and he held a telescopic high-powered rifle with which he shot people as they passed by.

I and the patient were able through this dream to flesh out an encompassing idealized image having the following features: (a) On the surface he was a meek and mild mannered, "Clark Kent." (b) Beneath the surface or at an unconscious level he was "Superman" or the superb sniper vindictively murdering or venting sadistic impulses toward all those persons who made his life oppressive, such as his nagging wife. (c) His migraines were his punishment for the existence of his sadistic impulses conflicting with his severe passivity and compulsive appeasement.

When Larry was able to work through the preceding three features of his idealized image, he could stand up appropriately to his wife and others, gain their respect, and do away with his "sniper" dreams. His migraines also went away.

Horney (1945, p. 116) suggests how the therapist needs to approach the patient's idealized image. First, the therapist must help the patient become familiar with all the facets of his idealized image. Second, he needs to aid the patient in discerning its many purposes and idiosyncratic standards. Third, the therapist must delineate the amount of misery it causes. Hopefully, the patient will then begin to realize in his gut that he is paying too high a price. However, the patient can only let go of his image if the primary requirements keeping it going are considerably weakened.

EXTERNALIZATION

Externalization is the tendency to feel that what you are really experiencing inside your mind is taking place outside and, generally speaking, to blame someone else for what you are feeling. As the conflict between the real self and the idealized image becomes greater, externalization enables the character disorder to turn away from himself. Externalization goes beyond projection in that not only one's faults but all feelings are experienced as outside.

Horney recognizes a little-known correlate of externalization, overdependence, that is, relying excessively on others for one's self-definition. Thus the patient focuses on changing others, punishing them, influencing them, rescuing them, etc.

Externalization induces a chronic sense of emptiness, shallowness, and drifting. When the character disorder experiences self-contempt, he may feel that others are looking down on him. Horney (1945, p. 119) advances the idea that the therapist should stay away from the negative aspects of the idealized image until the patient's despair is diminished and the idealized image is judged to be less in control of the patient. If the timing of the intervention is correct, the patient may begin to notice that his self-contempt is not grounded in reality but made up of his own personal, uncompassionate view he has of himself. A more compassionate attitude toward himself should increase the hope that his troubles can be surmounted. Externalizations are a formidable barrier to progress in therapy. Horney (1950a, p. 293) emphasizes that "Externalizations are the more difficult to recognize since they are often mixed up with his reactions to others on the grounds of his needs or the frustrations of those needs."

The following vignette depicts how externalization takes the form of blaming others for one's unhappiness, a misery really created mainly by oneself.

Laurie's overdependence on her husband and her need to avoid facing this trait fostered very evident externalization. Her husband was held by her to be responsible for causing her sense of abandonment and drifting propensities. She saw him as self-centered, caring only about money and his work. She felt, he did not make time for her. In actuality, Laurie had shifted her own narcissism to her husband. She did very little at home and indulged her appetite for jewelry through massive purchases on E-Bay. When her husband was available during normal day and evening hours, Laurie was asleep because she had remained awake during almost the entire night. She justified her strange waking and sleeping cycle by claiming that she had never been able to shift her former job's night hours to the normal wake-sleep cycle.

She was able to externalize her unconscious need to avoid intimacy by seeing her husband as refusing to stay up very late to keep her company.

She wouldn't accept his real explanation that he had to work the next day and drive a very long distance to his job whereas she could sleep throughout the entire day.

Rage, of course, can be directed against oneself as well as directed outwardly, as the next vignette demonstrates. The vignette also offers an instance where generosity subtly masks rage and/or anger at the same time. Horney (1937, p. 36) remarks,

> there is a marked contradiction between their wish for affection and their own capacity for feeling or giving it. Excessive demands concerning consideration for their own wishes may go with just as great a lack of consideration for others. The contradiction does not always appear on the surface. The neurotic may, for example, be overconsiderate and eager to be helpful to everyone, but if this is the case it is noticeable that he acts not out of spontaneously radiating warmth.

Florence's idealized image was that of the good little girl. This image compelled her to depend on others for their approval and gratitude as she compulsively did them favors. It did not seem to matter that the receivers of her favors were resentful and upset. They usually did not want her ministrations.

Her unwelcomed giving contained her externalized anger and the receiver's return of anger instead of expected gratitude represented her indirect savage attack upon herself. Florence was confused, lost, and depressed when her idealized image was not being verified. She kept redoubling her efforts to make her idealized image real so that she could be admired and cherished. She also directed her externalization of dependency and anger against her body. As a result she suffered from disabling attacks of asthma.

Externalization presents a number of significant difficulties in therapy. There may be a multitude of huge quandaries recited by the patient but she may be reluctant to examine and work them through. The patient may approach the conflicts in an intellectual or dispassionate manner. In this fashion the patient eliminates the authentic, feeling, real self. Horney (1945, p. 130) concludes that a patient who is not emotionally present will not be able to properly utilize any insight gained in therapy. He will not be able to apply his new comprehension to his life.

A byproduct of externalization is increasing alienation from the self. Horney (p. 117) comments that

> Another inevitable product of externalization is a gnawing sense of emptiness and shallowness. Again this feeling is not properly allocated. Instead of feeling the emotional emptiness as such, the person experiences it as emptiness in his stomach and tries to do away with it by compulsive eating. Or he may fear that his lack of bodily weight could cause him to be tossed about like a feather—any storm, he feels, might carry him away. He may even say that he would be nothing but an empty shell if everything were analyzed. The more thoroughgoing the externalization, the more the neurotic becomes wrath like and apt merely to drift.

The next vignette refers to the previously mentioned patient, Florence, a woman who suffered from episodes of asthma and utilized externalization.

Florence behaved as if there was no substance to her even though she had destructively attempted to gain a spurious significance through obesity. In treatment she seemed unable to apply any insights gained in therapy to life. She kept insisting through externalization that her husband must change before she could change.

IMPOVERISHMENT OF PERSONALITY

Horney wisely focuses on the havoc unresolved conflicts have on our functioning. They sap our energy, evoke inevitable frustration, point us toward the wrong goals, eclipse essential parts of our self, and hamper our creativity. As Horney (1945, p. 157) observed, "Waste or misdirection of energy can stem from three major disturbances, all symptoms of unresolved conflicts. One of these is a *general indecisiveness* [italics added]. It may be prevalent in everything, from trifles to matters of greatest personal importance."

One element of wasted energy is general indecisiveness; the following vignette is an example of this occurrence.

Leigh went back and forth regarding an appointment with a doctor to check out worrisome symptoms. During this period of extended doubt and repeated canvassing of her husband and myself as to whether she should go to a doctor, she wore out the patience of her husband and irritated her friends. She also had time to develop catastrophic fantasies of possibly having cancer or some other fatal disease. Consequently, she did not have much energy to do necessary chores, which also aggravated her marriage.

Another symptom of entangled conflicts is a general ineffectualness. Tasks take lengthy periods to complete and are done awkwardly or poorly. Inertia is a common feature, as the next vignette shows.

Leigh lay in bed and submerged herself in inertia. She expected her husband and daughter to do for her. When they objected, Leigh either sulked or raged against them.

According to Horney (1945, p. 160), "Neurotic inertia is a paralysis of initiative and action. Generally speaking, it is the result of a strong alienation from self and a lack of goal-direction." With regard to cause she said "Of the single contributing factors the most influential are the idealized image and sadistic trends."

Horney (1945, pp. 160–161) points out that having to exert effort to make things happen may be felt by the character disorder almost as insulting. He likes the idea of believing "If only I tried I could be . . ." This uncompleted action or merely an idea preserves his fantasy of potential greatness.

Impoverishment of personality leads to an impairment of moral integrity and egocentricity. Increased self-centeredness results in others being treated in a utilitarian manner. Horney (1945, p. 163) suggests that it is unthinkable to the character disorder that someone might not like him. He has to be admired or liked to preserve his self-esteem and reduce his anxiety. Others must be won over to increase one's self-worth. Others have to be blamed or defeated to avoid having to take responsibility for oneself. In some cases, others also have to be conquered to garner glory for oneself. Horney (1950a, p. 301) recognizes that "Sexual activities become not only a release of sexual tensions.

They can be a vehicle to drain self-contempt (in masochistic activities) or a means to act out self-torment by sexual degradations or tormenting of others (sadistic practices)."

The next vignette shows a patient using blame and externalization of her own wish to tease and flirt sexually with men.

Most men would notice Vicki. She dressed in a very seductive manner calculated to show off her enticing physical attributes. She once was hired by a car wash to parade in front of the establishment to entice motorists to notice the business. She wore a very skimpy bikini. Several car accidents were attributed to her distracting display. Despite her obvious physical attractiveness, Vicki was insecure about her appearance and her husband's continued interest in her as a desirable woman. When he undid his top shirt button, for example, she suspected that meant he was on the prowl, trying to capture the attention of other women. If he went to the gym, in her mind it was really a ruse to meet other women. She rejected all his denials of having an affair. She kept accusing him of potential infidelity.

The patient compulsively needed the perpetual adoration of her husband to allay her deep anxiety and self-hate. Vicki's love was parasitic and her proclamations of love were clearly a pretense of love. Her constant accusations and suspicions harassed her husband and made him a target for her sadistic impulses. She was entranced with the significance of surface and ignored the role of mother and wife. When confronted with her pretense of love in therapy, she would slip into a vacant stare followed by a hollow-sounding "I'm sorry." Needless to say her behavior did not change.

The next vignette portrays a patient who always thought of herself as on the side of the angels, or at least on the verge of being designated as a saint. She clearly illustrates Horney's concept of the pretense of goodness. Horney (1945, pp. 164–165) describes the false show as follows:

> unselfishness, sympathy and the like is akin to the pretense of love. It is characteristic of the compliant type and is reinforced by a particular kind of idealized image as well as by the need to blot out all aggressive impulses. Of course, the pretense of goodness leads to a depleted self.

Florence shoveled suggestions and solutions at others, whether or not they wanted her gratuitous counsel. Their irritation with her only temporarily deterred her. When she encountered resistance to her well-meaning efforts, she reacted with surprise, puzzlement and anger. She concluded invariably that she was a good person and that they were bad but they did not know it.

Horney (1945, p. 165) mentions other pretenses such as interest, knowledge, honesty, fairness, and suffering.

Unconscious arrogance is also a powerful disruption of the adaptive function of an individual. Horney describes this impairment as fueled by a sense of entitlement enforcing a demanding and devaluating attitude, which is buttressed by an assumption of supposed superiority. Horney (1945, p. 205) recognized the important role of the idealized image in maintaining sadism, grandiosity, arrogance, and entitlement.

She wrote about the character disorder "Since he himself cannot measure up to his idealized image, the partner must do so; and the merciless rage he feels toward himself is vented on the partner for any failure in this direction" (Horney, 1945, p. 205). Further "In reality he tries to enforce upon the partner the impossible task of realizing his—the sadist's—idealized image. The righteousness which he had to develop as a shield against self-contempt permits him to do so with smug assurance" (Horney, p. 205). Horney (p. 208) sums up the sadistic trend as follows: *"To be sadistic means to live aggressively and for the most part destructively, through other persons* [italics added]."

Explicit, exaggerated feelings of grandeur were displayed by the patient in the next vignette.

Sid based his arrogant demands and entitlements on his own sense of "correct," unchallengable assessment of "reality" heightened sense of "rightness." It did not matter that his wife and daughter suffered because of his egocentricity. There was to be no discussion or dialogue with them since there was no way he could ever be wrong. He issued decrees and they were to be obeyed.

I was seen harshly by him as naïve and muddleheaded. He was the only one with clear vision and therefore my strenuous attempts to invite him to try to make an effort to entertain a point of view other than his own were not to be trusted. The most difficult task for me during this phase of therapy was to keep my anger in check as I experienced his deeply rooted complacency about inflicting emotional stress on his wife and child. He ultimately dropped out of therapy after declaring to his wife that he had gone to a lawyer and was divorcing her. No amount of pleading on her part to continue working on himself in therapy would change his decision. He, of course, dropped out of treatment having issued what for him was another "correct" edict.

UNWILLINGNESS TO TAKE RESPONSIBILITY

Horney (1945) sheds light on another frequent aspect of the character disorder, which is the reverse of Sid's impairment. It is the inability to take a firm position and the undependability that is associated with it. The character disorder's conflicted emotional needs make decision-making erratic and flimsy. Anyone else's point of view may easily alter his own stand. As my patient aptly put it, "The last person who breathes in my ear, I follow." When they encounter the slightest difficulty in an undertaking they quickly give up and strive for a different goal. If the character disorder remains suspended between two choices of convictions, he may rationalize his undecided position by claiming that he is being indisputably fair or adopting what turns out to be a pseudo-objectivity wherein there is right on both sides.

Detached individuals may have the greatest objectivity but may have difficulty speaking or taking a stand. By contrast, the aggressive character disorder, for instance, whom we will meet in later chapters, can be decisive but is opinionated and dogmatic. His judgments are in the service of domination and recognition.

Horney addresses the issue of not taking responsibility for one's actions, an aspect of neurotic behavior that is present in all character-disorder impairments. Horney (1945, p. 171) defines taking responsibility for oneself as admitting to one's self and to others that you intentionally said or did something that was destructive and accepting the repercussions.

The next vignette is a dramatic example of a patient's unwillingness to take responsibility for his actions.

Tyronne was an ambitious entrepreneur, who cheated his clients and proudly removed himself from responsibility for defrauding them by announcing repeatedly to me "Caveat emptor" or "Buyer beware." He added "I didn't force them to buy my product."

Horney cites the diverse ways the character disorder tries to slip out of taking responsibility: denying, forgetting, belittling, feeling misunderstood or pseudo-retarded, convoluted rationalizations, and feeling unfairly accused.

The following patient reflects the narcissistic, expansive drive to control others and the spurious rationalization to continue her supposed reasonableness. The patient also shows the negative consequences of the narcissistic trend—the destruction of interpersonal relationships. Horney (1939, p. 96) writes about this aspect:

> The individual's illusions about himself and his peculiar kinds of expectation of others are bound to make him vulnerable. Since the world does not recognize his secret claims he often feels hurt and develops greater hostility toward others, becomes more isolated and as a result is driven again and again to take refuge in his illusions. Grievances toward others also may grow because he holds them responsible for his failures to realize his illusions. As a consequence he develops traits which we regard as morally objectionable, such as pronounced egoism, vindictiveness, distrust, disregard for others if they do not serve his own glory.

Betty was very angry with her son. She was very proud of her backyard garden and wanted her son to have his wedding there. He refused, telling his mother that his fiancée definitely wished to have the wedding in her neighborhood temple, a place she and her family had gone to since she was a small child. Betty summoned every argument she could to persuade her son and his fiancée that they were wrong, such as "The garden is more beautiful than the temple," and "I'm physically handicapped and it would be so convenient for me to have it in the garden," "If you really cared about me you would honor my request," and finally "I'm not going to go to your wedding if you do not have it in my garden."

I went over all her rationalizations and claims, pointing out to her that she was belittling her son and the bride's legitimate wishes. I added,

"After all it's their day, not yours." I tried to expose her efforts to induce guilt in them by citing her physical limitations which she was exaggerating. The patient responded to all my interventions with self-praise as a very "with it" person and besides that her son was under his future wife's thumb because he was going to have to sponge off her.

Her response to my interpretations reflected unshakable self-righteousness and smugness. Her idealized image was a declaration of super-sophistication and the arrogant entitlement to ignore her son and future daughter-in-law's rightful wishes. Betty was denying the consequences of her rigid, dogmatic behavior, belittling her son and bringing needless stress and suffering to what should have been clearly a joyous occasion. She was also expressing sadistic impulses under the guise of justice—really in thrall of a pursuit of a picture of glory as she imagined the wedding guests admiring her sophisticated garden.

Sadistic impulses, as in the case of Betty, will be discussed from the Horneyan perspective more extensively in the next chapter. Self-hate, tied so very closely to sadistic impulses directed by the character disorder against himself, will also be examined.

4 Sadistic Impulses and Self-Hate

SADISM

In the grip of hopelessness, the character disorder may give vent to destructive behavior. Horney carefully discriminated between assertiveness and true sadism. She recognized that it's all too easy to interpret sadism as appropriate assertion.

Horney required a pattern of sadistic expression before defining the patient's behavior as predominantly sadistic (e.g., a penchant for enslaving or victimizing others). The sadistic individual gives her partner just enough freedom to seduce him into continuing the dependent enslaving relationship. The sadistic individual advertises his unique positive attributes to convince her partner that he is in a privileged position of benefiting from his closeness to her. As the following vignette reveals, Horney (1945, p. 197) was well aware of the connection between sadism and exploitation. She observed the

> demands for special consideration, exclusive devotion, boundless tolerance. There is nothing specifically sadistic in their content: what does point to sadism is the expectation that the partner should, by whatever means that are available, fill out a life that is emotionally empty.

Betty made little effort to strengthen her weak legs. She also occasionally would lurch forward as if she was about to fall and her alarmed husband, in effect, had to remain closely glued to her side. He bitterly resented his virtual imprisonment enforced by his wife's presumed physical impairment. He rightly sensed that his wife was exaggerating her infirmity (a slew of physicians had established that there was no organic basis for her impairment) and could do a lot more than she displayed. He would erupt periodically into rages, then return to a guilty, submissive role to indulge his wife's manipulative dependency.

Betty was able to express her underlying anger toward her husband for his rigidity (e.g., he would insist on doing garden chores in a wasteful, unvarying manner despite Betty's clear explanation to him of a quicker, better way to complete his tasks) by cramping his chance to live a freer and happier life during his retirement years.

Betty illustrates a number of characteristics of the sadistic character disorder. She clearly played on the feelings and needs of others and/or frustrated their wishes. Betty also used guilt-producing behavior to manipulate her husband, because there was no way he could even think of momentarily separating from her because she appeared so presumably helpless and physically disabled. Horney (1945, p. 197) captures the essence of sadism, observing that its most common feature is not mere ungiving but a purposeful yet unconscious awareness of the extensive need to frustrate the other—to destroy their legitimate hopes and aspirations.

With regard to the sadistic character disorder, Horney (1950, p. 209) notes that

> If he can convince himself that he is entitled to exploit or frustrate them without their complaining, criticizing, or resenting it, then he can keep from becoming aware of his tendencies to exploit or to frustrate. If he is entitled to having them *not* [italics added] expect tenderness, gratitude, or consideration, then their disappointment is their hard luck and does not reflect on his not giving them a fair deal.

The sadistic person is very good at employing various means of humiliating and disparaging others, as the next vignette shows.

Douglas knew his wife felt bad about her obesity and in every argument he would inject a vile comment about her weight and tell her she was not at all sexually appealing. When his wife wanted to discuss finances he would impatiently dismiss her questions as stupid. On occasion he would ask her what she wished to do on a weekend, then abruptly reject any of her choices. When they were out with another couple, he would scornfully contradict her comments and in general communicate to their friends that he did not regard his wife as in any way intelligent.

Douglas had attained great professional success. He prided himself on his exactitude and demanding standards, qualities demanded by his profession. He applied his perfectionistic attributes to other areas of his life. Anything he purchased, for example, had to pass through a rigorous multitude of tests before he made a decision to buy it. No one in his home, his wife included, was permitted to touch anything of his without his permission. If he thought his wife or daughter had dared to touch one of his possessions or even move an item belonging to him one millimeter, they were subjected to a vicious trial of accusations and questioning.

He would occasionally disappear in the evenings, leaving his wife without any means of reaching him despite his having a cell phone. To his wife's repeated requests to leave his cell phone on so that he could be reached in the event of an emergency, he retorted firmly "I don't like to be called." His attitude in general in and out of session was quite simply "If I tell you something and you think it's unfair, you do not have the right to question me." When his wife informed him that his young daughter had been very hurt and humiliated when he criticized her speech in front of her friends, he just shrugged his shoulders and retorted, "I do not see anything wrong with correcting her grammar in public when she makes a mistake."

Horney would probably see Douglas as able to rationalize his sadism as honest and helpful. Through externalization and distrust of anyone else's possible adequacy, he disparaged his wife's and my feedback. Horney (1945, pp. 198–199) describes Douglas' attitude quite well. She sees someone like him as disparaging any person who is offended or hurt by his mistreatment. He will dub that individual as overly sensitive or weak emotionally. The capacity to be concerned with someone else's feelings was absent in the patient and he could readily express contempt toward his wife whom he depicted as emotionally unstable. Douglas once told me that my thinking was deficient or very pedestrian and not in the same league with his own superior, uniquely different thinking. I asked him at that moment to consider why he took so much pleasure hurting my and other people's feelings. His response was to stare at me in silence while his whole posture conveyed disdain and seething scorn.

The cause of sadism or the creation of sadistic trends, Horney conjectures, is a profound futility regarding the character disorder's own life. The sadistic patient is convinced that he can not change his life for the better. Envy is one outgrowth of this bitter resignation. He feels deprived of the good that others seem to possess. As Horney (1945, pp. 201–202) indicates, the joy or happiness of others and their mundane pleasures annoy him. "Why should they be happy," he thinks, "when I am not?"

Concomitants of bitter envy, according to Horney (1945), are a "sour grapes" attitude, fault finding, devaluating, vindictiveness, and a constant feeling of disappointment and discontent. Despairing of ever being able to reach his excessive standards the sadistic character disorder is taken over by self-loathing. Any criticism of him brings on overload and he rejects the feedback as unfair, undeserved blame. He then desires to humiliate the critic through externalization. Horney (p. 205) puts her finger on one interpersonal outcome of envy when she notes that, failing to fulfill his idealized image's standards, the sadist relies on his partner to compensate for that failure by succeeding. If the partner does not attain the prerequisite success she deserves anger and vitriolic condemnation, the same feeling the sadist has toward himself.

It should be mentioned that Horney (1945) does not acknowledge that she is following in the footsteps of the pioneering English analyst, Melanie Klein. Horney resided for a time in England before coming to America. She also sent her children to Klein for a brief period of analysis. Klein first enunciated in a lecture her conviction that envy played an important role in neurosis in 1924 in a paper titled "An Obsessional Neurosis in a Six-year Old Girl." In this paper Klein connected frustration with envy and sadism. She linked the origin of envy to a primal scene exposure. Klein emphasized the central role of envy in her treatment of her 6-year-old patient. She (Klein, 1975, p. 56) wrote "This envy proved to be the central point of Erna's neurosis."

Melanie Klein through further clinical experience extended our understanding of envy and another attitude, gratitude, detailing the nuances of these two aspects of character in her book *Envy and Gratitude* (1975).

She saw envy beginning early in life, perhaps within the first year of life. Putting aside Klein's highly speculative notions about the infant's supposedly sophisticated mental functioning, her discussion of attitudes triggered off by envy can fit nicely into Horney's model of character trends. Klein sees envy as essentially spoiling the emotional life of both the envious one and the one who is envied. The envious patient begrudges the therapist's good work, thus avoiding a feeling of gratitude. Strong envious feelings can destroy the patient's capable cognitive functioning. Envy can cause rageful attacks upon the partner followed by doubts as to whether the sadist is really a nice person. As a result of enviously attacking the therapist the patient may become overwhelmed by guilt or anxiety, feel both discounted and deprived of therapeutic nourishment, and greedily cling to the therapist. If the patient could regain a greater capacity to love and express gratitude, Melanie Klein asserted, envy would decrease along with anger and feelings of persecution.

Horney, like Klein, ties the formation of envy to despair culminating in rage and sadistic behavior. She notes that the sadistic character disorder feels strength and pride when he distributes pain to others or causes suffering. He is worried or frightened that the therapist will take away his sadism which equals power and he will become a contemptible "worm."

The world is perceived as threatening and anxiety-producing by the sadistic character disorder, who must remain hypervigilant out of fear that the world will treat him in the same destructive manner as he mistreats others. Horney (1945, p. 210) cautions the therapist to first help the patient to become aware of his sadistic proclivities. This is a difficult task, because the patient is so good at rationalizing or denying any sadistic proclivities that he even fools himself into believing he is kind and gentle.

Each character type rationalizes sadism differently. The compliant type enslaves the partner under the guise of needing love; the aggressive type justifies his sadism as being in the service of honesty, and with the belief that his victims deserve the treatment they receive. The detached character disorder expresses sadism in a more subtle way, stealthily frustrating the needs of his partner through omission or withdrawal or inducing guilt.

If sadism is very repressed, the character disorder is overly constrained and timid. The individual does not risk expressing a different point of view or speaking up against abuse. She may even oppose her own needs for fear of offending. To avoid the emergence of anxiety, the character disorder places "handcuffs" on the satisfaction of legitimate needs and, as Horney (1937, p. 55) points out, the "inhibition goes so far as to check awareness of its existence."

The following vignette dramatically highlights the almost unbelievable lengths a character disorder will go to not to hurt another's feelings.

Sherry was on the phone with a friend. The conversation had gone on for about an hour and she was feeling a strong, increasingly insistent urge to urinate. She feared that her friend would be offended if she terminated their conversation. Sherry instead stayed on the phone and urinated into her clothes.

The character disorder who has repressed sadism will move heaven and earth to avoid offending or embarrassing the other, even at their own expense, discomfort, and suffering.

Burying sadistic urges can lead to increased self-hate and self-contempt, which results in part from timidity and susceptibility to victimization. The link between sadism and self-hate, a central feature of Horney's theory, was elaborated by her in her final major book *Neurosis and Human Growth* (1950a).

THE ORIGIN OF SELF-HATE

According to Horney, self-hate begins when the vast gap between the idealized image and the real self creates a feeling of failure, a sense of being a bluff and an object of contempt. The process of self-idealization is accompanied by pride, which sets the stage for the creation of a basic deep conflict between the pride system and the real self. In effect, there is a huge battle between healthy and neurotic forces which results in the dichotomization of self-idealization and self-hate, and globally a huge battle between healthy and pathological forces.

THE FEATURES OF SELF-HATE

Self-hate is tenacious and powerful and the patient continues to feel the self-hate in everything he says or does. Adding to the tension and anxiety, the neurotic is alienated from his real self and is persecuted by his own arrogant standards. Pride in whatever the patient feels or does blinds the patient to the self-destructive, self-hating aspects of his behavior and prevents him from taking responsibility for the self-hate. Horney (1950a, p. 116) suggests that the essential content of the process is frequently externalized, that is, seen as if other people hate, dislike, and/or do not respect the patient instead of the patient registering that he is the one who really hates himself. Horney (p. 118) lists six manifestations of self-hate: (1) compulsive mandates on the self, (2) unforgiving self-accusations, (3) self-contempt, (4) self-frustrations, (5) self-torments, and (6) self-destruction.

Horney (1950a, p. 118) introduces the concept and role of the "shoulds" (the "have to" and "musts") and their relationship to self-hate. The "shoulds" are caused by self-hate and pride. Vehemence, always residing in self-hate, is also freed when the patient is not in touch with self-hate's presence within him. Therefore he is unable to reduce or control it. In addition, morbid dependency is fertile soil for self-hate to grow. The excessive need to cling to another individual as a rescuer or super-protector without regard for their qualities weakens self-respect and fosters self-hate. Finally, there is the "should" which mandates perfect behavior or the necessity of accomplishing every impossible goal.

The following vignette illustrates a patient's futile search for glory by entering into a relationship that clearly promised from the start definite self-punishment and increased self-hate. A conviction of invulnerability accompanied by dreams of a glorious relationship also seduced the patient. Horney (1950a, p. 34) comments "He needs to feel invulnerable— and behold! his imagination has sufficient power to brush off pain and suffering. He needs to have deep feelings—sympathy, love, suffering: his feelings of sympathy, suffering and the rest are magnified."

The patient, Burt, knew very early in his relationship with Harriet that she was mean and that she was treating him with contempt. Her own best friend had warned him not to marry her. But Burt, admiring what to him seemed her successful, courageous resistance to her dysfunctional family and moved by sympathy for her past traumas, ignored these distinct warnings. He subsequently married her. Nineteen months later the patient had one child from this clearly destructive marital union and was involved in an intense custody battle with a now alcoholic and promiscuous ex-wife.

Burt's chief defense was alienation from his self. He had cut himself off from his initially healthy, severe, self-preservative inner misgivings and allowed himself to function on automatic. His life had now been turned into a chronically vexing ordeal resulting in complications that would burden him for a good part of his life.

His self-hate had a number of childhood origins. There was first his "innocent" (his term) mother, and second a self-hating, alcoholic father who had suicided when the patient was 18 years old. Burt had built his self-hate along two conflicting, self-destructive character trends: the naïve attitude of his mother and the self-hating, impulse-ridden behavior of his father.

Burt's predicament illustrates some basic concepts of Horney. His self-hate, for instance, mandated that he rescue his wife from her pathology. This powerful urge drove him into an obviously destructive relationship. His "should," namely that he succeed, was too powerful for him to discard. Then too there was the tantalizing prospect of obtaining glory if he indeed did rescue his seriously emotionally damaged wife. Probably at an unconscious level he sensed that his wife would inflict suffering upon him, but his idealized image reassured him that he would be invulnerable to her painful attacks on his self-esteem. How best to treat Burt given all the unhealthy forces maintaining his self-hate?

I first challenged his despair that he could never change his life for the better by focusing on his self-hate. I wanted him to experience the full totality of his self-hate as an aspect of his character structure. I had come to the conclusion that Burt's real self was sufficiently strong enough to weather the greater awareness of the magnitude of his self-contempt. I struggled along with him to reduce his alienation from his self-hate. During this alliance of mutual therapeutic effort I employed various metaphors to alert him to his ongoing program of self-created suffering. I asked him to consider the possibility that his efforts to rescue his wife and passive compliance with her narcissistic wishes were akin to lowering an empty bucket into an empty well or trying to pin jello to a wall. It looked easy and could give the patient the illusion of possibly actualizing an idealized self's sense of triumphant glory. He volunteered in so many words that he had thought that he should be able to tolerate unlimited abuse. What remained to be uncovered was his hope of doing the impossible and the delicious pride and arrogant grandiosity that would follow.

At a certain point in therapy, just when it seems that the self-hating patient is on the verge of really making progress, the negative therapeutic reaction (NTR), a recrudescence of symptoms, may set in. Horney (1936) was the first analyst to fully explore this puzzling and frustrating phenomenon in therapy. The basic cause of NTR, according to Horney, is the dawning realization of the patient that he has realistic limitations and is not able to accomplish everything he desires. As Horney (1950, p. 120) puts it, "These realizations, mostly unconscious, make him panic because he feels he *should* [italics added] be able to overcome all these odds."

To prevent the eruption of self-hate, the character disorder resorts to a number of defensive measures. He may work at not being aware of his self-hate, or he may experience life as acting upon him instead of perceiving himself as the author of his life. Basically self-hate is being driven by an unfulfilled "should," that is he should not be self-hating as long as he is convinced at bottom that he is a superhuman being.

Horney (1950a) is convinced that pride, an invariable element in self-hate, plays an important role. The character disorder, failing to reach the pinnacle of success, intelligence, power, is subject to an indictment by his pride in or out of therapy. The exposure of a neurotic problem appears to him a dreadful sin. He may attack himself or perceive others as looking down upon him. A vicious cycle is set in motion. The character disorder having fears loses his conviction that he is a god-like being and losing this special status intensifies his self-contempt and fears.

He may fear that he will be discovered to be a fraud. What he fears most are his pretenses: pretenses of love, fairness, interest, modesty, and competence.

The following vignette reveals the impatience the character disorder feels when his search for glory is not quickly satisfied. He also experiences a surge of self-hate in the form of not letting in any good that is offered to him. This clinical example demonstrates how the character disorder tries compulsively to give himself some modicum of self-esteem. Horney (1987, p. 85) refers to "the various kinds of prides, self-idealization itself, of the insistence of being accepted by others, on being useful to others and so forth."

Calvin was respected and looked up to by members of his therapy group. He deserved their respect because he consistently was empathic and able to powerfully transmit his compassion and insight to the other patients. He was not, however, compassionate toward himself and frequently stated that he felt like a fraud waiting to be exposed. The group was alternately puzzled, confused, and on occasion angry with Calvin's tenacious hold on his definition of himself as a fraud. It was only later on, when he started a new job and immediately expected to have the same power as the president of the company, that both the group and I gained a more complete insight into his idealized image.

Apparently a feature of his idealized image was the pretense of nuanced fairness to others, such as the group and therapist, but beneath this was the arrogant claim that he was superior in competence to everyone at work and in the group. Therefore, he expected, even claimed, that the president of the company would recognize the reasonableness of his claim. Calvin expected the president to consult with him before making any significant decision. At the same time he was afraid that they would ultimately spot this arrogance and he would be fired. He had been let go from jobs in the past but he had always presented his dismissal plausibly as the company's problem.

On a deeper level he also was concerned that he was not as competent or special as he would like to believe and ultimately he would be found out. For a time Calvin used the exploration of his self-hate and its connection to the fear of exposure in the service of further fault-finding with himself. This self-hating process had to be repeatedly brought to his attention so as to turn him toward a constructive use of his increased knowledge of the destructive consequences of his idealized image.

Horney (1950a, p. 126) points out that the above-described patient does not get his priorities straight or see the pertinent details so as to deal properly with a social situation. Certainly this was the case with Calvin, who also verifies another observation of Horney's. He had trouble accepting any feedback concerning his obvious strengths. He would respond with: "You only said that to make me feel good about myself," or "You are the therapist; that's what you are supposed to say." The same reaction held true for feedback from the group when they told him how intelligent and perceptive he was in his participation in giving insight to any member of the group.

Horney (1950a, p. 126) observes about certain patients that they may agree that the therapist's intervention is correct, but inwardly they have made a reservation that the therapist is probably wrong that or what he said to them was to make them feel better. The "should" that is active here is the unrealistic conviction that there is no situation or problem that he could not handle or should not be able to handle. As if postulating an Euclidian geometry theorem, the patient, Calvin, failing to resolve anything he wished for, thought he was the most vile creature on the face of the earth. He leveled upon himself every base accusation and reproach. His self-hating dynamism was a "damned if you do and damned if you don't" paradigm. About this vicious self-hating cycle Horney (1950a, p. 129) notes that the patient is bent on reinterpreting his actions into a negative view of himself and turns things around. If he aids another, he is a sucker. If he doesn't come to someone's rescue, he is selfish. Complicating and retarding the positive consequences of an interpretation is the patient's readiness to link the intervention with his proclivity for relentless, crushing self-accusations. Therefore, he readily embraces guilt, counterattacks, or blames someone else.

Horney (1950a) describes various consequences of self-contempt, namely, comparing oneself adversely with others; a compulsive need to attain the impossible, that is, superior competence in every area; vulnerability to criticism; accepting too much abuse from others (e.g., Burt, who passively complied with his alcoholic wife's wish to have a child and his acceptance of her promiscuity); and finally an excessive need to seek admiration and approval.

Depending on the character type various aspects of the self are despised. The aggressive vindictive character disorder will despise whatever he believes is his "weakness."

Horney (1950a) introduces the concept of self-limiting taboos: taboos negating enjoyment, taboos prohibiting spontaneity, conflict, happiness, growth, hope, and aspirations.

Self-hate may cause the character disorder to be self-destructive. Horney (1950a, p. 151) presents the idea that the patient engineers his relationships over and over so that he can be punished by his friends, spouse, and family members.

The following vignette is an example of a patient who caused members of his family to distrust his future behavior because of his flagrant, destructive acting out in the past. It also shows how this same patient could not understand why certain family members took reasonable precautions to protect themselves from his possible acting out. What made it difficult for the patient to understand was the patient's alienation from his self. He was one of those many character disorders, according to Horney (1950a, p. 156) "who live as if they were in a fog. Nothing is clear to them. Not only their own thoughts and feelings but also other people, and the implications of a situation, are hazy."

Bob's drinking and drug use caused him to be unstable at times and not likely to be a responsible and suitable usher in the wedding party of his cousin. His past self-destructive acting-out was well known to all the members of his family. His aunt, the mother of the bride, fearing an emotional scene, chose not to include him as an usher at her daughter's wedding. This rejection was experienced by him as an unforgivable, humiliating blow to his self-esteem and, from that point on for more than 20 years, Bob punished his aunt by not speaking to her and not attending any family function where she just might be present. He took great pride in "getting even" with her although his vindictive retaliation also punished his wife and broke his mother's heart.

Bob is a prime example of Horney's observation that the character disorder attempts to make others, in this case his aunt, the author of his fate or victimizer of him. He ignored and/or denied that he was responsible for his aunt's legitimate apprehension based on his past behavior. He also did not accept her many apologies.

ACCEPTING ONLY THE GOOD

Wenkart (1955), a Horneyan analyst, suggests that accepting only the good and not the bad leads to non-acceptance of the self. I would add that it perpetuates self-hate. She offers the following example of a patient, Lucy, who is very distressed over having pimples on her face. Lucy felt a compulsive urge to scratch and rid herself of what she thought was a horrid blemish.

Wenkart (1955, p. 138) quite rightly points out, "As we are not made of alabaster we do have pimples at times." She further states that "The angry scratch, the revengeful squeeze, aggravate the healthy condition. We have to accept the healthy and the unhealthy, the pleasant and the unpleasant. We have to accept conflicts."

A line from a poem by Walt Whitman (1861, p. 92) is quoted by Wenkart as an example of a healthy view of conflict, of polarities, of contradictions: "Do I contradict myself? Very well then I contradict myself (I am large, I contain multitudes)."

The next vignette depicts a patient who had every material and seemingly every emotional need met yet because of excessive claims and an intolerance for the vicissitudes of aging, she fumed and spoiled any good she was receiving.

Every invitation I offered to the patient to entertain a wider view of her life, of the good that obviously existed in her life, was emphatically rejected. As Horney (1987, p. 82) puts it "This means that he believes himself always to be right." Horney (1957b, p. 181) also suggests that the therapist keep in mind about the patient. "Is it real suffering that he can learn something from or neurotic suffering that he uses to disguise vindictiveness, to provide alibis, or to serve as a basis for claims?" "Finally, he may falsify his affects and believe that he suffers when actually he is filled with rage."

I visited May, an elderly patient, at home in response to a request for a consultation by her devoted son. When I arrived at her home it was quite clear that the patient was surrounded by wealthy, loving, and successful adult children, with two live-in attendants whom she could order to satisfy her frequent whims. I witnessed her in a royal manner commanding them to fetch and satisfy her frequent wishes. She had recently undergone surgery and was recovering nicely. Nonetheless, she railed against her age and her physical limitations. "I hate myself!" she cried out.

I could not reach her because, as Wenkart (1955, p. 141) writes in accordance with Horney's model, " A patient does not know that he is harming himself. He is all self-hate and nothing of him is left to sympathize with the mistreated self."

There is a lovely parable attributed to the Buddha that addresses the need to have compassion for oneself, a concern that the patient, May, did not exhibit. A grief-stricken mother comes to the Buddha because she is stuck in anguish at losing her young son. The Buddha quietly listens to her touching lamentation, tells her to take a seed, and instructs her to give up this seed when she encounters any family in the nearby village that has not suffered some major suffering or misfortune. When she returns she tells the Buddha that she still had the seed because there was not one home she visited that did not experience some terrible tragedy. She could now begin to move past her own pain, that is, to sympathize a lot more with her beleaguered self by recognizing that suffering and/or loss is an inevitable part of life. She had not been specially singled out for a unique misfortune.

The next vignette shows how a character disorder may set up such high, unreasonable standards for acceptance of a possible good that self-hate is then reinforced and spuriously validated. In effect, the patient in this clinical example tried to achieve her goal of a close relationship with a man, as Horney (1950a, p. 212) observed about many expansive character disorders, "by compelling fate through the height of their standards."

Julie felt anxious and empty when she did not have a serious relationship with a man. Her previous relationships always ended when she found the men unexciting both physically and mentally by her own perfectionistic criteria. She entered therapy when she began to recognize that she was too dependent on an unrealistic fantasy of "love."

Julie described how she was always scanning men and asking herself "Is this the right man?" or "He's cute. I wonder if he is the right one?" This constant scanning caused her to have butterflies in her stomach and tension.

In therapy we explored how Julie did not really feel lovable and this conviction led her to wonder if any man could ever love her. Self-hate was expressed through the belief that she was unlovable. She began to recognize that she really desired a "superman," one who would love her and end forever her doubts about her own self-worth. Each man had to be tested to determine whether indeed he was the truly perfect, strong man who would rescue her from her self-hate. At the same time her per-fectionistic filters made the chances of a "good" man coming through to her real self very slim if not impossible.

The next vignette illustrates how an adaptive defense against anxi-ety, anticipatory functioning, can become perverted into a powerful in-strument of self-torture. Anticipatory functioning can increase self-hate when it is linked to the tyranny of a "should." Horney (1950a, p. 65), for instance, points out that the character disorder believes "He should know, understand and foresee everything." She (Horney, p. 74) refers to a patient who "was very proud of what she considered her gift of foresight and of preserving her family from dangers through her prescience and prudence." But she failed to anticipate correctly one time. The result of this failure was that the patient "felt as if the ground had been pulled away from her" (Horney, p. 74).

Worrying about the future is rather commonplace in our society and can even have a salutary function as a way of preparing us for contingen-cies. No doubt our primitive ancestors saved their lives on numerous oc-casions by asking themselves, "What if a wild beast is lurking behind that bush waiting to pounce on me?" Since we must all be survivors of that ancestor we all carry within us a penchant for realistic and unrealistic an-ticipatory propensities or worry. Obsessive, morbid worry is adaptive anticipation gone astray as the patient, Donna, exemplifies. Horney (1937, pp. 268–269) comments about individuals such as Donna, writing, "the neurotic unconsciously exaggerates his weakness and he tenaciously insists on being weak," and "Patients may imaginatively seize upon every possibility of believing they have an organic illness."

"You would have thought I would be very relieved when the doctor told me I did not have cancer. I was for a minute; then I began to worry about some other part of my body going haywire." Donna said this with a puzzled

expression. "I keep tormenting myself with worries like will I be able to handle the next surgery I have to have?" The patient had begun her morbid worrying from the time she was 13 years old; that was the moment her hair had begun to fall out and she had to deal with her own feelings of mortification, shame, and humiliation. Her peers did not help her get through this painful time. They jeered and ridiculed her appearance. Some boys even took cruel delight in calling her derogatory names and physically abusing her. More trauma followed. When she was 18 she lost her father to a sudden heart attack. Her mother developed a strange, fatal illness that could not be diagnosed and ultimately she died while Donna was in her early 40s.

In the session to be described I was again faced with Donna's unrelenting self-torment in the form of compulsive, catastrophic worry. At one point in the session I asked her if she had ever felt any modicum of compassion for her besieged self. She hesitated and in a somewhat bewildered voice answered "No!" She did remember, however, that she had shown compassion and maternal protectiveness toward her 13-year-old daughter when she had been taunted by a peer. "So you could be protective and compassionate to your daughter but never to yourself," I said. There was a long pause. I could see from her facial expression that she was thoughtful and deeply affected by my statement. She then said "Yes, but why don't I care about how I pick at myself now? Where is my compassion?"

My intervention had momentarily liberated her from a "should" that was unmercifully tormenting her real self. She now had the option of taking a more potent role in demanding increasing self-caring concern for her victimized real self. She had been seduced into thinking that morbid worry equaled compassion and concern. She had also identified with her adolescent tormenters and become a persecutor of her suffering self. With her beginning wonder in therapy a door had been opened, leading to possibly more appropriate self-compassion away from self-contempt.

THE CHALLENGE OF BRIEF
HORNEYAN PSYCHOTHERAPY

It should be recalled that once-per-week psychotherapy imposes great, almost insurmountable challenges (Bocknek, 1993; Kelman, 1945) to the therapist to somehow touch upon those issues that matter or should matter to the patient. The Horneyan model has within it enough of the most significant elements frequently present in the character disorder, such as self-hate, "should," claim, etc. These aspects offer the Horneyan therapist a good opportunity to help the patient toward emotional health.

The following is a general ground plan that the Horneyan therapist follows as much as each patient's dynamics will allow. It should be noted that Karen Horney's model of treatment is not ambitiously and unrealistically perfectionistic.

Just as the artist paints a general outline, the Horneyan therapist draws out the character structure of the patient and the genetic details. Thus, therapy should be an attempt to delineate the main character trends: their consequences, self-hate, "shoulds," claims, prides, and the relationship each character trend has to the other. Finally addressed is their interconnections with the encompassing idealized image.

Centering mainly on the present symptoms, I believe that the treatment of the following patient illustrates the applicability of the Horneyan approach within once-per-week therapy to the problem of self-hate and sexual acting-out. Working within the Horneyan approach facilitated my understanding of the patient and the patient's understanding of himself.

Charles, a 30-year old unmarried man living with his widowed mother, was sent to me by the county probation department because he had exposed himself in public. This had been his first lapse, which occurred on the same day that he had learned of his failure to pass an examination for appointment to the position of county policeman.

He had committed the offense while mildly inebriated. He freely admitted that he had driven his car to a remote neighborhood and exposed his genitals to a young housewife who was working in her front yard.

Riddled with feelings of inadequacy and self-hate, he exposed himself in order to affirm his masculinity. From another point of view, his public act of passion carried within it the expectation of his being loved for himself—his hoped-for assertive, real self. Confounded by the consequences of his own unique set of claims and "shoulds," wracked with self-contempt, and misguided by a particular idealized self-image, he was rendered passive, self-alienated, and impotently enraged. He desperately needed a sudden magical solution. Despite its adverse consequences, his loss of control was a germinal, misdirected act of emancipation. It had been precipitated by his keen yearning to free himself of his inadequacy and self-hate—a yearning which overwhelmed even his fear of losing control.

At the beginning phase of therapy he worked through some aspects of both his inadequacy and his fear of losing control. A homosexual advance made upon him accelerated his confrontation with his fear of losing control. Instead of going berserk as he feared he would, he merely pushed the man away. The incident illuminated his chronic anxiety about destroying people, and the interpretation was given that, despite the provocation and his fear, he hadn't killed anyone. As a further consequence, his compelling "should" to hold back all intense feelings was revealed. Extreme feelings were tantamount to dangerous impulses. In perceiving this he could then experience how the "should" had punitively cramped his feelings and obstructed his relationships.

Emerging next was the issue of his passivity, which was related to his feelings of inadequacy and self-hate. His passivity was supported by the claim that his mother's obvious depression and isolation be ameliorated without any effort on his part. Interconnected with this claim was the "should" that he put up with his mother's negativism and defiance: he should tolerate, for example, that his mother would not answer phone calls, that she would go about in tattered clothes—shaming him before the community—and that she would not obtain a needed hearing aid despite his repeated requests that she buy one. Exploration revealed that he had not really confronted her decisively about any of these irritations.

His lack of forcefulness had intensified his inadequacy and self-hate and betrayed evidence of his prides and his idealized image. He was constrained to show the world that he was a compliant, self-effacing, dutiful, well-controlled, all-American son. Therefore, he should not get angry when his mother screamed at him or abused him. There was pride in not wanting anything in the way of intimacy for himself. He became more aware of a conflicted need for closeness which his pride in the simple pleasures of life had defended him against. His simple pleasures were shown to be superficial attempts to gloss over his feelings of loneliness and detachment. Thus, a typical social week consisted in playing ball and drinking beer with the boys.

Now more cognizant of the wants of his real self, he dreamt that he saw a group of people lifting a car off a pinned man. This was interpreted as showing a constructive need to assert himself, to face his trapped feelings, not to quit on life, and to retrieve his oppressed real self.

Experiencing his profound self-alienation, he tearfully expressed his guilt and his sorrowful disappointment in his family. He felt his loneliness, sadness, isolation, and self-effaced yearning for love. But his despair was lightened by my expressing admiration for his heartfelt confirmation with feelings that he had warded off for years. He was told that he was beginning to take down a wall between himself and others—a strong, constructive first step in reducing his cramped self-control, alienation, and inadequacy.

With regard to his developmental history, Charles as a child had repeatedly witnessed drunken battles between his mother and father. Hovering on the sideline, he fearfully watched his mother provoke his father into beating her. This loss of control by his father was internalized by Charles so that he feared that he would become angry enough to beat women. At the same time he identified partially with his mother and set up situations in which he would be beaten by life. For example, his genital exposure and the exposure of his license plate, driven by self-hate, conspired to assure his apprehension by the police. His self-control was in response to a fear that he would hurt himself or others, mainly women, through masochistic or sadistic assaultive behavior respectively.

Charles also felt a sense of impotence when he saw that father's beating of mother did not halt her berating him. Father could not reach mother, just as he had trouble altering her behavior now.

He was able to connect his fear of losing control, his sense of inadequacy and passivity, to a series of childhood incidents in which he was abused or infantilized by his mother. When he was young, his mother had continually called him her baby and had loudly shouted in the streets a term of endearment that withered him. "Bube" was the term, and Charles associated it with breast. He sensed that his inadequacy was appended to a fantasized image of himself as an extension of his mother. Lacking in autonomy, he felt passive like a baby before all women. And as a baby he was unable to have any adult, mutually intimate relationship with any woman.

At one time he had been assertive and unafraid of women. He remembered that during the latency period he would occasionally hit his mother in response to her chronic taunting and belittling. Guilt feelings sharply curtailed this trend toward assertiveness, and through reaction formation he became piously contrite, attending church regularly. This was the beginning of his self-effacement and his confusion between being aggressive and being assertive.

Contributing to his inadequacy was an experience during his adolescence. A girlfriend learned of his mother's term of endearment and embarrassed him by repeating it. This later turned out to be a memory contributing to a deep-rooted belief that somehow he was dirty to women. He had transferentially divided women into two categories: one, the idealized mother, unsullied and virginal, who was not to be approached by him; and, two, the dirty, polluted mother who could not be touched because of a threat to his pride system. Evidently his mother would curse and swear at his father, so that Charles could readily transfer these "dirty" qualities to women. The result of his intense ambivalence was detachment, isolation, and a sense of inadequacy and/or self-contempt in the presence of all women.

Since therapy is still ongoing, childhood recollections of inadequacy and of wanting emotional contact with mother are continually emerging. He is going through a process of mourning for the mother he never had but wanted and for the father he had cherished and despised.

5 Valid and Invalid Claims

In most instances a good dictionary is best when it comes to defining a term. However, in the case of the concept "claim," as Horney employs it, synonyms are most suitable to portray all the nuances of her theoretical view. The following are an array of synonyms for the term "claim" (Rodale, 1978, p. 171): right, request, demand, challenge, appeal, plea, and pretension. And so it is with the meaning of Horney's "claims," which can range from a relatively mild request to a demand and even a supplication or plea. As Horney (1950a) uses the concept of claims to elucidate character pathology, she focuses more on the patient's invalid demand for special treatment by the world. But in a sense, as we shall see, a patient's claim can embody all the symptoms above, some obvious, others less so. Claims serve at times to defend, protect, or obtain gratification of needs on demand. The defensive and/or protective value of a claim becomes similar to a "cage" that can also be thought of by the "caged one" as a safe refuge. To the patient, abandoning her cage (Connelly, 2002, p. 262) can be a terrifying experience. The therapist's challenging task is helping the patient dare to leave her prison to discover a better life.

What is a claim in Horney's schema? It is the righteous expectation that a wish or desire deemed valid be gratified immediately or later. Claims can be valid, realistic, and healthy or unrealistic and unhealthy. Examples of healthy claims are the expectations that traffic lights function properly, that police appropriately enforce the laws, that people make some attempt to understand us, and that a significant other consider us a priority in his or her life.

Unhealthy claims or entitlements are the following: Expecting one's suffering to justify for inappropriate, manipulative control; expecting that emotional and/or physical pain can be inflicted on another and he or she should endure the mistreatment; expecting not to age; expecting that one could eat vast amounts of food, not exercise, and not get obese; expecting that one's health will always be excellent; expecting not to ever lose a loved one; expecting that one will invariably be liked and admired; expecting that one will always be free of conflicts, doubts, anxieties and sadness; assuming that one's life will be forever joyful; and feeling entitled to a spouse who never gets upset.

Claims or entitlements emerge as a pervasive and significant aspect of our daily activities. Horney (1950a) focuses on the consequences of an excess and misuse of claims.

Probably, entitlements originate as a function of childhood suffering. An individual may believe that he or she is special or different from others. Narcissistically, an individual may assume that he or she has the right to treat or be treated by others in a privileged manner because of the way he or she once was suffering or indulged, the way he or she still is suffering or pampered, or the way he or she will be suffering or tormented. Claims are not always pathological. In relation to his parents, for example, a child has the valid right, short of perfection, to have his physical and emotional needs optimally met.

The significance of claims is illustrated in the following segment of a therapy session:

Harold and Shirley entered the room and immediately sat far apart from each other. In his usual obsessional, systematic fashion, he said that he had taken some notes concerning events that had recently annoyed him in their marital relationship. Becoming angry, Shirley countered by denouncing him for being self-centered and ungiving. She added that she wanted another house as their present one was too cramped and embarrassingly small. Harold felt that this was not the best time to purchase a home since their marriage was "rocky." Again, Shirley saw his hesitation as another sign of his unwillingness to give to her. Harold in turn perceived his wife as never being satisfied and not registering all the positive moves he had made, such as taking her into the city on her birthday. Previously he had dreaded and phobically avoided any trips into the city.

What are the claims in this confusing array of accusations, counter-accusations, and mutual discontents? Harold felt entitled to a total forgiveness that would erase all his past sins of self-centeredness. He also felt entitled to be complimented for those moments when he had shown some growth. Shirley felt entitled to attack him because "one swallow does not make a summer." She also felt entitled to lash out at him because, by not buying a larger house, he demonstrated to her his lack of change and his lack of commitment to her needs. During the session Shirley manifested the entitlement of not having to look at her own responsibility for the rift between them, such as holding on to her anger. She merely repeated her grievances, seeing them as totally justified.

Further illustrations of the role of entitlements in therapy are in the following segments:

At 28 years of age, Robert came into treatment because of marital difficulties. As he put it, "My bubble burst, and I discovered I really didn't have the good marriage I thought I had." Strengthened by therapy, he began to challenge his wife's persistent coldness toward him and her need to intimidate and manipulate him. As his own self-esteem increased and as he felt more "manly," he felt a wish to end his marriage to his erratically warm spouse. Robert yearned to be the carefree bachelor. There was only one hitch: he still had considerable doubt that a divorce would bring him superb joy. If he stayed in his marriage, he reasoned, perhaps it could become better.

His claim to safety, no matter what choice he made, was revealed by his use of a metaphor: "If only I knew that at the end of the tunnel of my marriage there would be light." My response was, "Unlike the usual tunnel, Robert, finding light depends upon the attitude with which you enter the tunnel."

His entitlement of prescience stemmed from his being reared in a dictatorial, Prussian-like atmosphere where no dissent was permitted. In such a home everything was ordered, and the future was a smooth extension of the past and present.

His use of "tunnel" describes aptly how claims are like "mind tunnels" or "cages". They enclose our thinking and feeling sometimes, as in the case of valid claims, leading to light and increased positive options or, as in the case of Robert, directing us toward darkness or restricted, negative, self-destructive consequences.

The following vignette exemplifies the virulent, destructive power of pervasive self-hate and claims and how the patient, Vincent, through therapy won release from his imprisoning entitlements.

When I first met Vincent at the community mental health clinic I was reminded of the chronic, "picked off the street," burnt-out alcoholics.

He was living with his widowed mother who wanted him to leave. He had nowhere to go, having lived in his car for a month before his mother relented and allowed him to stay with her. Every day, he claimed, his mother taunted and insulted him, calling him "lazy, a good-for-nothing and a defective."

The patient experienced a wide range of feelings in response to his mother's bitter accusations and persistent scolding. A predominant feeling was murderous rage: "I would like to choke her."

Vincent related to me in an obsequious, self-effacing manner. He would nod agreeably as I offered him my understanding of his self-destructive claims, particularly the entitlement to have others magically take care of his needs without him doing anything other than bathing in self-pity. He felt that he had been abandoned and placed in his perilous financial position when he lost a lucrative job obtained through his father. This loss of job and death of his fearsome, ambivalently protective father buttressed his claim that the world should somehow recompense him for this traumatic, unfair loss.

It seemed that his father had been a middle management Mafia enforcer, a gorilla type who thought nothing of lunging at a man whom he thought offended him and punching him in the face. Like the patient's mother, the father openly devalued the patient and would challenge him repeatedly to be a "man" like himself. This meant coming at the father physically and subduing him. The patient never challenged his father on this score.

As a young child, Vincent frequently witnessed his father reach across the dinner table and smack his mother across the face because she dared to ask him why he was out with his latest whore the night before. As a child the patient never could understand why his mother risked questioning or arguing with his father when the result was always the same—a quick, brutal blow across her face.

What confused him even more was his mother's fawning behavior toward his father at other times. He concluded and still believed that she was and is a "phony," a sly woman who venerated just one thing—money.

Vincent's father both despised and was frightened by the timid passivity existing in his son and controlled his fear by abusing the patient. Evidently, the father's unverbalized claim was that the patient had to be an even more intimidating creature than he was and rise to the top of the Mafia food chain since he, himself, would never make it to the Godfather status.

Excessive eating and general neglect of his health led to the father having a fatal, massive heart attack. The patient's fearsome and powerful protector was now gone and the "sharks" moved in. One day four Mafia "soldiers" entered his office and quietly and firmly suggested that he resign from his lucrative, cushy post or else.

Vincent would frequent bars and would easily succeed in convincing a woman to invite him to live with her. Ultimately, the woman would become frustrated, tired of supporting him, and ask him to get a job. He would fail to find employment and would be asked to leave. He would then feel entitled to rage at the woman, accusing her of betraying him and, on occasion, physically abusing her. He would, of course, be thrown out on the street and back he would go to his mother. She, in turn, would not welcome him but continue her tirade against him, and his own disappointment in himself and his self-hate would reemerge in full force.

He then usually halted his drinking and substituted a familiar refrain instead: the claim that he had a right to self-pity because his father was no longer around to protect him and hand him a good job.

It was very difficult to like Vincent. I particularly felt an aversion toward him when he described how he had smacked a woman because she dared to "mouth off" at him. He was proud of his forceful and "manly" way of showing her who was boss. I linked this entitlement to his father's physical mistreatment of his mother and him. He did not care that his mother was hit, saying "She deserved it," but he was able to finally relinquish this entitlement when he thought again of how terrified he felt when his father went after him. He still saw women as mere objects to be used, was verbally abusive to them, but no longer wanted to physically assault them.

He revealed that he had tried many times to initiate some truly innovative, creative social programs in a union, but they were squelched by his father. The father, we perceived, had been threatened by the possibility that the patient was superior to him in creativity and organizational ability. Once Vincent realized this he was able to challenge his destructive, necessary demand that his father had to be invincible and superior to him (i.e., he needed this perception of his father as "superman" to suppress his desire to compete with him. Competition might result in a devastating reprisal by his father). He could give up his magical dream of glory and launch a realistic program of constructive progress. He enrolled in a city college and was able to graduate and obtain a job. He had also met a very intelligent woman, Martha, who financially supported him, evidently seeing the patient as a "diamond in the rough." He admired her great capability and was able for the first time to care about and give to another human being. Where once he had adamantly told me he would never marry, he did marry Martha.

I realized that the description of Vincent's therapy may sound like a fairy tale that went along quite smoothly. Such was not the case. There were many blockages, many derailments. First, there was the claim of self-pity, already mentioned, to overcome. Second, there was his running away from responsibility for changing his life. Then there was his entitlement to treat women as his father had dealt with his mother. Later, there was also his transferential distrust of me where he suspected and accused me of despising him. There was his own self-hating externalization of his self-hate, defining him in an image of uselessness, inadequacy, and hopeless dependency. At first he also did not dare to express any anger toward me until he was able to trust that I would not excoriate or physically abuse him the way his father did.

Vincent had another unappetizing trait. He was bigoted and would pridefully express his prejudices, particularly against Afro-Americans. Paradoxically, he saw them as violent, even as he imagined explosive, preventive, threatening scenarios with himself as the indomitable hero. I presented this contradiction to him and asked him to consider that what he hated and wished to subdue or annihilate existed within himself. In other words, Vincent relished persecutory fantasies from minorities, distracted himself, and defended against his own self-hate. This intervention gave him pause and caused him to wonder seriously how much he saw the world in general in a highly personalized and distorted fashion.

According to Horney (1950a, p. 41), claims require that "Everyone ought to cater to his illusions. Everything short of this is unfair. He is entitled to a better deal." Every claim is the result of an egocentric justification. Vincent, for example, was not fully aware that his claim and entitlement, the right to strike women, was really striking at his rejecting mother. He was aware of his claim to be taken care of by a woman, but he justified it and his self-pity based on his childhood suffering and present financial privation. He at first expressed his bigotry claim and justification for it based on some threatening experience he had endured in a slum where minorities resided. His illusions were: all women were like his mother and he could strike at them and reject them; and all minorities were a physical threat to him. Horney (1950a) emphasizes the basis of claims. The claim embodies the disparity between the reality of being an individual with the expected human frailties and the wish to be a super-human being. The claim becomes a demand that this disparity no longer should exist. It is as if the patient is saying, "I want this to be, therefore it is." Grandiosity plays a role here, asserting the steadfast conviction and proud question put to others: "Do you know whom you are talking to?" The response that is expected is, "You are a very special person entitled by destiny and superiority to be treated with special consideration, attention, understanding, and respect." One patient, for example, wondered why a teacher was annoyed with him when he asked her to start the class 15 minutes later because he had a hard time getting to the class on time. He was angry at the teacher, whom he saw as not considerate of his needs. This patient illustrates the finding that, if the claim fueled by a wish is not fulfilled or is denied by others, the frustration of that wish and claim is not acceptable and is unjustified. The offender deserves to be punished.

Horney (1950a) gives examples of patients voicing a range of common claims: the woman who expects that her doubts about herself would be erased by a loving and doting man; patients who are convinced that they are never wrong and how dare anyone criticize them or offer a different viewpoint. Then there are those patients who feel entitled to con others and cheat them, such as the patient, Tyronne. Finally, there are those patients who claim that their bodies never age or suffer an illness, that entertainment always be first class, and that no test ever be given to them. Once claims come into being, arrogance enters the arena. With arrogance comes fragility and distrust in the possibility that anyone could possibly like them, love them, or think they are adequate. A common saying of the patient is, "There must be something wrong with any club that would have me as a member."

The following segment depicts how a claim of unlovableness prevents letting in love.

Jim could not believe that his wife loved him despite her repeated declarations of love for him. He could not let in her love because he claimed not to be very lovable. The more his wife proclaimed her love for him, the more he distrusted her. He also did not want to be ruled by the necessity of what he saw as an unfair claim to return her love. He saw this as a dictatorial entitlement of his wife and he was determined to fight her on this just as strongly as he fought his father's truly unjust claims on him. She wanted him to change and he felt entitled not to change, a defiance of a basic demand of the universe that nothing ever remains the same.

Another component of claims is envy. Envy at bottom is an outcome of a claim, the entitlement not to be who one is but to take away an admired possession or trait of another. The therapist is often tasked with an assumed pact, "You, the therapist, are to help me attain what I envy most, a perfection."

Claims also mean exceptions, such as, "Others have to work, not I," or "If I am in financial difficulty, I must be given money to bail me out," or "I can be successful without making any effort," or "I can be fuzzy about what I want and it will not matter," or finally, "I can be passive and the good things in life should somehow come to me."

In therapy, the patient, Horney (1950a) notes, presents a list of demands that the therapist must fulfill. This becomes a one-sided contract, as the following segment depicts:

Ivan emphatically stated when asked by me to enter a group, "Why should I? You are supposed to change me. That's why I come to you." Told that the group might help him recognize more clearly his rigidity and immense anger, he responded with a counterclaim allocating to himself a greater mental health stability than members of any group. This claim entitled him not to listen to them or respect their possibly valid feedback, such as, "They are more likely sicker than me. Why should I listen to them?"

A common claim is one where the patient may minimize the role of his blockages in determining how successful therapy can ultimately be in releasing him from his defensive, self-created "cage," such as, "You are the therapist. You should be able to get past my defenses. There must be something wrong with you. Just how competent are you?" The patient then feels quite comfortable in further expressing discontent and irritability toward the therapist. The patient may vindictively demand a sacrifice or payback from the therapist to right the scales of his or her neurotically defined concept of justice. On the part of the patient this amounts to the following, "I do not take any responsibility for change. You, the therapist, should succeed anyway. Since you failed, I am owed special compensation."

Horney (1950a) stresses that vindictiveness is always present along with claims in character disorders. The justification for the existence of entitlement is the patient's past and present conviction of special suffering and the general unfairness of life. Vindictive claims are actively and aggressively asserted. They are seldom expressed timidly to others as well as to the therapist. When the patient, for example, shows impatience, he displays an unwillingness to tolerate suffering. By frequently disagreeing with opposing viewpoints or the therapist's interventions, the character disorder asserts the entitlement to have the world ordered exclusively to his needs. If he is foolhardy, he reinterprets his behavior as brave, epitomizing solid self-esteem.

To support the validity of a claim, the patient exaggerates his contribution to the therapeutic process. This may be merely bringing his body to the session, braving inclement weather, being a loving person with good intentions, or paying the therapist's fee. Horney (1950a) suggests that rejecting the patient's claims only works when the individual himself is demonstrating some authentic signs of assuming responsibility for himself.

The character disorder may idealize any good he possesses, perhaps referring to having given at some time to others, to substantiate the validity of his claims. It is a tilted bookkeeping schema always in favor of the patient as creditor and the therapist as debtor.

The idealized image, "shoulds," pride, the solutions all serve to keep the character disorder going. By "solution" Horney (1950a, p. 186) means character trends that have an encompassing, pervasive effect throughout the self. She states further that

They give form and direction to the whole personality. They determine the kinds of satisfactions which are attainable, the factors to be avoided, the hierarchy of values, the relation to others. They also determine the kind of general integrating measures employed. In short, they are a *modus vivendi*, a way of life.

Claims, part of the solution, can be forcefully presented as an obligation to be fulfilled, a mandate based on justice, suffering, pity, compassion, love, and self-sacrifice, or they can be supported by irritability, harsh confrontations, and guilt-producing statements.

Sometimes a claim can be based on a promise, as the following vignette shows.

With respect to promises as a supporting determinate of claims, Bill would promise to be more loving to his wife. The promise would then be converted into a claim, an obligation that she would in turn be more loving and forgiving of his infuriating passive-aggressivity. Once his wife forgave him, he would then revert back to sulking and irritability. She would become angry again, confront him, and Bill would rear up in righteous indignation, saying, "How dare you become upset with me. Didn't I promise that I would be more loving?"

My attempts to have him see how he was "gas lighting" her, a process used unconsciously to drive a spouse "crazy," met at first with little success. My efforts ran up against another powerful claim and blockage, such as, "I'm such a nice guy. I wouldn't do that to her." I retorted, "But you yourself told me that sometimes you like to get even. Is that nice?"

Claims that are all-encompassing cause chronic pessimism and discontent. Character disorders only notice what is lacking or differences, not the good that is there. They become easily disgruntled with any unfamiliar, new situation. Trivial upsets are converted into monumental distress. They do not, in common parlance, "go with the flow," "take the unforeseen in stride," or "roll with the punches." As one patient once recalled, "I had had it. Getting a ticket was the last straw." He had parked in a clearly marked illegal parking space, an action stemming from his claim to be above the law. He said, "I looked up at the sky when I saw that ticket and I screamed 'God! Why are you pissing on me?' I didn't care who heard me."

The patient who indicted "God" is expressing envy, according to Horney (1950a, p. 59). He is convinced that bad luck is his lot alone. He is being especially singled out to be persecuted and he envies everyone who to him lives a life singularly free of any problem such as loneliness, panic, or cramping limitations, including receiving a ticket.

Given the character disorder's premise, that is, "I'm entitled to anything I wish," he may be puzzled as to what in truth he really deserves. He lacks that reliable conviction as to what is right or wrong and muddles along, giving vent to sometimes outrageous claims.

The following is an example of an outrageous claim:

Roger, the patient, and his friends had finished lunch. His friends had left tips for the waitress next to their plate. Roger discovered that he lacked a dollar so he reached across the table in a nonchalant manner and removed a dollar from a friend's tip. His action was noticed by a friend who had remained behind. He confronted Roger with his inappropriate action, saying that the waitress would wrongly think that she had not been tipped properly by the friend whose dollar was now in Roger's hands. He could not accept that he was doing anything wrong. His claim was quite simply, "I don't have the required amount. My friend does so I have the right to take from him." He complied with his friend's rebuke and put the dollar back.

It took many, many sessions and many incidents before the patient finally got it. He was able grudgingly, with great reluctance, to experience how his self-righteous, narcissistic claims offended others. Roger always felt it was right to express claims with certainty. If a thousand people told him he was wrong, he would still charge ahead with invalid entitlements. I had to repeatedly recite to him a Persian proverb, "If two people tell you you are a horse, get a saddle," to puncture his arrogant self-centeredness and bold proclamation of his unhealthy claims.

Since claims are often not backed up with the requisite effort to make them real, the character disorder is frequently unhappy, depressed, and fatigued. It takes a lot more energy to keep asserting unhealthy claims that will never be fulfilled than to exert the required effort to make the goals of valid claims realizable.

When claims are not met, the character disorder blames everyone but himself. He says "If only I had been helped." But more than being helped, what he wants is to be fixed. And why not? He would have to challenge the whole array of claims he lived by, if he initiated effort. His whole *modus vivendi* would have to be given up. Horney (1950a, pp. 60–61) points out that the character disorder may go through a series of intricate, defensive maneuvers, such as, "I don't have any claims," "What are you talking about?" "Okay, I do but they make sense." Finally, "Big deal! Let's talk about something more important."

Magic is always the court of last resort. There is the conviction that willpower will conquer all. Employing magical thinking, the character disorder stays on course, convinced that ultimately his claims, no matter how unrealistic, will definitely be gratified. He believes he has a secret deal with fate and sings to himself the refrain "wishing will make it so."

One patient, Tyronne, used to make up lists of claims and after each one he would carefully inscribe "And so it will be done." To him this inscription insured that his entitlement would absolutely come true. He believed that his specialness endowed him with supernatural power or, should we say, he had a desperate need to validate the inordinate demands of his idealized self.

The character disorder is engaged in a lifelong "lottery" and his claims are his lottery tickets. He lives as if he will ultimately grab hold of the "gold ring," and then fame and glory will be his. Why work or deal with temporary frustration to build a realistic future. So what if realistically life has become more narrow, devoid of true attainments; his entitlements will continue to endorse his grandiose illusions about himself. In the meantime, he wants the world to conform to his righteous demands. He does not want to recognize that his entitlements are really a plea for fulfillment of magical glory and, if he can attain some insight into the unrealistic trap he has labored to create, he will then truly become a "prince" (i.e., a "prince of a fellow") rather than remain a "frog." (i.e., a mediocrity).

6 "Shoulds," Glory, and Pride

"SHOULDS"

The chapter heading, "The Tyranny of the Shoulds," in Horney's book, *Neurosis and Human Growth* (1950a), introduces an essential component in her theory. Horney postulates based on her clinical experience that the character disorder

> holds before his soul his image of perfection and unconsciously tells himself: "Forget about the disgraceful creature you actually *are*; this is how you *should* be; and to be this idealized self is all that matters. You should be able to endure everything, to understand everything, to like everybody, to be always productive"—to mention only a few of these inner dictates. Since they are inexorable, I call them "the tyranny of the shoulds" (Horney, 1950a, pp. 64–65).

"Shoulds" are rules, commands, mandates, and decrees unconsciously dwelling within the self. They are inescapable. As maxims they tell the character disorder what he "should be able to do, to be, to feel, to know—and taboos on how and what he should not be" (Horney, 1950a, p. 65).

What are some of the specific characteristics of the inner dictates, that is, the "shoulds"? The individual is to never feel insulted, sad, tormented, or anxious; he should always be unruffled and/or spontaneous. "He should know, understand, and foresee everything" (Horney, 1950a, p. 65).

"Shoulds" do not care whether goals are doable and display "a complete *disregard for the conditions* under which they could be fulfilled" (Horney, 1950a, p. 66). A "should" may demand that the individual should always be empathic and compassionate, whether or not he actually has these traits. "Shoulds" are convictions that nothing is impossible to be or do.

The character disorder, living a good part of the time in her imagination, will eradicate any limitation or weakness. Horney (1950a, p. 70) cites a patient who became aware that she had a huge drive for power. The next day she became convinced that this drive belonged to the past; consequently "She should not be power ridden; so she was not" (Horney, 1950a, p. 71). Horney (p. 71) recommends that the therapist help the patient recognize that "shoulds" can not be erased by a magical effort of will power. Will power attempts may be an attempt to rapidly protect against an upsurge of feelings of weakness and defeat.

"Shoulds" may appear as "I should be able to master, for example, depression, guilt, daydreaming, impotence, and disgust with myself." On occasion the patient may externalize her disgust with herself and instead imagine the therapist as being disgusted with her.

"Shoulds" can be applied to almost any aspect of life, such as, "I should be getting away with anything" (Horney, 1950a, p. 73).

There can be conflicting "shoulds," (i.e., self-preservation versus masochistic rescuing) such as the "should" to be an ideal supporter of an alcoholic husband. Sometimes a patient's self may become almost fragmented, verging on the edge of a psychotic break. The patient, dimly aware of the inner tyranny of a "should," may adopt three possible attitudes toward them: mastery, love, or freedom.

Some consequences of various attitudes toward a "should" are: self-righteousness, crushing guilt, rebellion, passively conscious or unconscious irritation, hypersensitivity toward coercion, and listlessness. "Shoulds" have an array of consequences: a feeling of effort, impaired interpersonal relationships, damage to feelings, pseudo feelings. "Shoulds" may evoke prohibitions against tenderness, empathy, anger, and hostility. Horney (1950a, p. 85) concludes that

We cannot in fact understand the full impact of the shoulds unless we see the extent to which they are intertwined with self-hate. It is the threat of a punitive self-hate that lurks behind them that truly makes them a regime of terror.

The following vignette illustrates the formidable power of "shoulds" to cause stress and have compulsive, self-hating consequences.

Arthur endured intense pain in his heels. This tormenting sensation proved puzzling until his basic "should" was understood. Apparently, the patient watched tensely every facial expression of his boss. He scanned his employer's behavior for every sign of approval or disapproval of job performance. He dreaded being fired and this fear caused pain in his heels and disabling headaches. Mondays were especially difficult since Arthur struggled through Sunday evening with the terror that his imperfection in the form of incompetence would be discovered by his boss and co-workers. He felt that he literally had to walk vigilantly on tip toes. He felt he should do so to preserve his emotional safety and job.

In the grip of "shoulds," other people are perceived as having the same "shoulds" as the patient. Consequently, the individual heartlessly criticizing himself imagines that other people should find him wanting in some particular way, as in the case of the preceding patient, Arthur.

"Shoulds" influence our capacity to be aware of our feelings or how we express them. A character disorder may think that he is spontaneously experiencing a feeling when he may merely be displaying the behavior that the "should" mandates. Non-genuineness or pseudo-feelings are a consequence of the pervasive power of the "shoulds."

The following is an example of the interaction between "shoulds" and a lack of authenticity.

Vicki, the very "sexy" patient discussed in a previous section, was constantly accusing her husband of being attracted to other women and wanting to have an affair with them. If a waitress wore a low-cut dress and a miniskirt, her husband's glance at her confirmed for Vicki that he was on the verge of making a date to have a sexual liaison with the waitress. No amount of declarations of love for the patient by her husband seemed to reassure her.

Vicki was in the grip of an overwhelming, relentless "should," namely that her husband should have his eyes glued totally on her. He should also always return home on time and fire any female employee who dressed provocatively as defined by Vicki.

Her "shoulds" were destroying her marriage, forcing her husband to say repeatedly that he felt as if he was in a prison and Vicki was his jailer. She would summon forth a pseudo-feeling of indignation that her husband would even consider that he was being persecuted when she was the one who was going to be betrayed by an unfaithful spouse. On occasion, the patient would become contrite and issue an apology, but her accusations of infidelity would shortly return, continuing the marital disharmony.

"Shoulds" can be created to enforce what are on the surface wonderful attributes such as love, generosity, and sympathy. A character disorder may be mandated by a "should" to be the utmost of generosity, love, and sympathy, but in truth these mandates enforced by "shoulds" become ersatz or cosmetic and have no genuine authenticity.

We discover how shallow the "shoulds" of perfect love are, for example, when we see how quickly love turns to hate or disappears or becomes indifference.

There are "shoulds" that compel ruthlessness or vindictiveness. There are "shoulds" that are camouflaged with high-sounding rationalizations.

The following is an example of a couple which illustrates how a "should" could bend their morality so that they could accept deceitful, harmful treatment of others.

Tyronne and Gina could easily express disdain for anyone who lost their money to Tyronne's make-believe business schemes. They would say "This is a dog eat dog world" and they were just being more "realistic" than the average person.

Here is another example of various "shoulds" contradicting each other, forming a coalition of painful conflicts.

At the drop of a hat April would list all the emotional atrocities perpetuated upon her by her husband during their 35 years of marriage. He criticized her appearance, housework, and job. If she brought home news of a promotion from her boss, he would disdainfully say, "So what! You are in a job where they are so desperate for help, they would hire anybody."

April felt she should accept the pain meted out to her by her husband. Contradicting her desire to escape from his pain, April felt she should not have to listen to any suggestions from family or friends as to how to extricate herself from a hopelessly intolerable marriage.

The following is another example of the deleterious consequences of a "should."

Barbara was in a bad relationship with a man that had lasted for 7 years. Though she had a good job and earned enough to support herself, her fear of loneliness kept her in a frustrating, conflicting turmoil. One "should" proclaimed that she remain with her angry, rejecting boyfriend because she at least was familiar with his limitations. The other "should," a healthy one, announced that she should leave quickly and begin finding another apartment.

As a child, Barbara was told by her mother that she should never have been born, that her existence burdened her mother's life. Barbara had dealt with this malignant "should" by countering with another "should," one which mandated that she not allow herself to feel or desire. This "should" numbed her so that she did not feel the pain of her mother's rejection, but it caused her to feel that she did not exist, satisfying in a way her mother's wish. The patient's "should" also prevented her from reaching out and obtaining a good relationship with a mature man. She felt that she was not entitled to feel or certainly not to feel good. She was to suffer like her mother suffered from desires that were never met.

Malignant "shoulds" continue from childhood to adulthood unless we become aware of their existence and reliably and tenaciously remove them.

The following is an example of a malignant "should" inflicting pain on a patient.

Ronald believed that with continued effort he could finally win some sign of his father's love, although throughout the patient's life, his father had consistently shown the absence of any affection, tenderness, or approval toward him.

One particular incident tellingly portrays the father's severe limitation. Ronald had searched long and hard for a suitable birthday gift for his father that would particularly please him. He placed the gift in front of his father's usual chair the morning of his father's birthday. He, of course, was certain that this time when his father saw the present he would be obviously appreciative and grateful to his son for the great thought that must have gone in to selecting the gift. Instead, his father sat down with the gift in plain sight in front of him, slowly ate his breakfast without saying a word, and as he got up to leave the table he turned to Ronald's wife and thanked her for the thoughtful gift. Nothing in the way of gratitude was subsequently said to Ronald. He was treated once again by his father as the "invisible" son.

Though Ronald was a law-abiding citizen, by contrast to his younger brother, a member of a motorcycle gang and an eager participant in barroom brawls, apparently in his father's eyes Ronald was not "man enough" as his younger sibling was to gain his father's respect. The father's message was that the patient should have been a boxer, as the father was in his younger days, or an inebriated street-fighter; then he would be loved. Confused, Ronald retreated into martial-art video games and excessive overeating. Ultimately he became quite obese and diabetic. He appeared to be on his way to fulfilling his father's wish, that he should not exist or that he should kill himself, since he was not completing his father's idealized expectation of masculinity.

A particular "should" may occupy so much of our mind that it may become terrifying to give up. Such was the case with Rhoda, the patient in the following vignette.

Rhoda was involved in an affair with a married man, who was much older than she was. Her own marriage was very unsatisfying, but she felt she should (the first "should") remain in it because her parents had divorced when she was a child and she had vowed never to duplicate what she saw as traumatically shattering to a child. Her relationship with her lover was stressful and frustrating. One moment he would tell her he loved her and the next instant he would coldly inform her that he had business to transact and would be gone for a few months. Although Rhoda vowed to end the affair, she was terrified to endure the empty space the unsatisfying affair filled. She would back away from saying a permanent goodbye to her lover. She felt she should (second "should") be able to change her lover's mind so that he would treat her reliably well and even leave his wife.

Rhoda entered group therapy and was repeatedly confronted by the group members with her self-destructive relationship with both her husband and her lover. She responded by threatening to leave the group because they should (third "should") be more sympathetic, empathic, and compassionate to her plight, and they further should (fourth "should") come up with a novel tactic to either free her from her lover or better yet change him so that he would leave his wife and marry her. All these preceding "shoulds" prevented Rhoda from accepting any insights into her own self-frustrating behavior and the discovery of how much she was captured by her malignant "shoulds." She seemed determined pridefully to accomplish the impossible and continue to endure the obvious mistreatment by her lover and herself.

A word about the use of group therapy. Although Horney (Rubins, 1978, p. 274) was interested in this modality and even tried it, she ran into major difficulties in her application. The technique was too unfamiliar to her. As Rubins (p. 274) states, "Each patient was relating and reacting not only to her but to the others at the same time. Each was reacting differently to her. And their reactions were not the simple, understandable ones she had anticipated. It was like juggling six balls in the air at once." Horney ended up somewhat skeptical about the value of group therapy in the treatment of patients. Still she wished that the technique would be studied further and "encouraged setting up a research study project in group psychoanalysis at the Institute in 1945" (Rubins, p. 274).

My own experience with group therapy in the treatment of character disorders suggests that it can be a valuable supplement to individual psychotherapy. Of course, it will not work with every patient. Nonetheless, with many character disorders the multiple feedback of individuals in the group can go a long way in reducing blockages and encouraging responsibility for one's own behavior.

GLORY

"The search for glory" delineated by Horney (1950a, pp. 17–39) is expressed in an individual who

> wants to express his idealized self, to prove it in action. It infiltrates his aspirations, his goals, his conduct of life and his relations to others. For this reason, self-idealization inevitably grows into a more comprehensive drive which I suggest calling by a name appropriate to its nature and its dimensions: *the search for glory*. Self-idealization remains its nuclear part (Horney, p. 24).

According to Horney (1950a) there are a number of crucial elements that lay the groundwork for the search for glory. It may be an early childhood home where there is chiefly an absence of reliable love because the caretakers are too egocentric. This leads to basic anxiety, defined by Horney (p. 18) as a "feeling of being isolated and helpless in a world conceived as potentially hostile." Basic anxiety results broadly in three possible moves. The individual may become excessively dependent on the most forceful person around him; he may become defiant and oppositional; or he may draw a "wall" around himself and become guarded. The moves may contradict each other and their clash constitutes the basic conflict. Characterological solutions such as compliance, expansiveness, and detachment originate from the basic conflict.

Conflicts drain self-confidence and cause a divided self riddled with inhibitions. Feeling angry and separated from others, the character disorder is driven "to *lift himself above others*" (Horney, 1950a, p. 21). The character disorder strives to obtain safety and to obtain this goal he subdues his real self containing his genuine goals and wishes. He becomes alienated from his real self, his feeling of identity. He creates through imagination an idealized image to give himself power and importance.

What does the character disorder idealize? He glorifies "his particular 'solution' of his basic conflict" (Horney, 1950a, p. 22). He dresses up the solution with camouflage so that aggressiveness becomes assertiveness; detachment becomes self-sufficiency; compliance becomes cooperation.

Horney (1950a, p. 123) observes that "Once the character disorder identifies with his idealized image . . . he becomes this image: the idealized image becomes an *idealized self.*" Horney introduces another concept, the comprehensive neurotic solution, a construction devised to gratify all the inner needs, a self-realization to make the idealized self a reality.

To accomplish the idealized self, the character disorder engages in a search for glory through various means: a need for perfection; compulsive ambition; striving for power, popularity, admiration, and deference.

Horney (1950a, p. 26) devotes her attention to a singular destructive aspect of the search for glory, namely *"the drive toward a vindictive triumph."* The goal of vindictiveness is to either shame or vanquish the other through achievement.

The search for glory is characterized inevitably by compulsiveness, a "must" rather than a spontaneous desire that is indiscriminate (e.g., he must be the center of attention no matter what the situation). The search for glory is insatiable, with acute feelings of frustration when it is thwarted. According to Horney (1950a, pp. 34–36) the character disorder's imagination works overtime fabricating potentials as actual attainments, promising unlimited possibilities and, for example, unlimited knowledge. Recognition of limitations is prohibited. In essence glory-seeking is seeming and fantasy, not being and truth (Horney, pp. 38–39).

The drive for glory leads to a nonacceptance of limitations or responsibility for negative treatment of others. Blaming others becomes a frequent occurrence. The following is an example.

Betty, the patient who pressured her son to be married in her backyard garden, had a problem with her legs requiring a wheelchair. Her immobility did not stop her from carrying out her chief dedication to glory. This was her need to control everyone around her. She was quite adept at doing this. By means of the telephone and various catalogues, she was, for example, able to manipulate and persuade various companies to give her special treatment. She also had her husband scurrying about carrying out various tasks mandated by her.

When her son was about to be married, she requested that he have his wedding in the garden of her home. Both her son and his fiancée had decided on a wedding in a temple that had a special significance to the prospective bride. Betty unrelentingly pressured her son to comply with her wishes, ignoring her son's and future daughter-in-law's clear and strong wishes. Betty assembled a whole host of reasons that to her justified having the wedding in her garden. All her reasons were obviously self-serving and elicited her son's anger. That did not matter to Betty. She was bent on absolute control and, in keeping with her search for glory, appropriate reality considerations were irrelevant or worthy of being ignored. She did not attend the wedding, creating a lasting bitterness in her son and spoiling the happiness of the newlyweds.

The search for glory may manifest itself in less obvious ways, as the following segment depicts.

Roberta, for example, restricted her search for glory to a subtle competitiveness with colleagues. A favorite tactic of hers was to begin a question aimed at a co-worker at a staff meeting in the following manner: First, she would praise the colleague for his astuteness or valuable contribution; then she would insert a "but" and proceed to demonstrate the foolishness of the idea.

Roberta felt compelled to be the center of attention, the most intelligent and the most valuable member of the firm. As Horney (1950a) points out, the search for glory is compulsive, an absolute "must." Roberta sabotaged her own good self-interest, illustrating another observation of Horney. The patient was disliked by her co-workers. They struck back at her through petty, obstructive actions, making her work that much more difficult than it had to be.

The next example of the search for glory is on a personal note.

When I was much younger and filled with more powerful drives for professional success than now, I spent long hours in my office in the basement of my home. There I studied the psychoanalytic literature, wrote papers, and saw patients. One evening my 8-year-old daughter, Leigh, knocked on the office door and asked me if she could play at being a patient. I thought at the time that her request was charming and I entered into her childish "let's pretend" game.

It was only much later, thinking about our pretend play, that I recognized that my search for professional triumphs was blinding me to what really mattered. I was not in touch with a reality. My daughter was giving me a message, attempting to summon me back to my family, to pay appropriate attention to her legitimate emotional needs and not sacrifice these needs on the altar of glory. She intuitively sensed that only as a make-believe patient could she possibly wean me away from the dazzling splendor of unrealistic glory to discover what really mattered—involvement with my family.

The pursuit of glory can create self-doubts and self-destructive conflicts, as the next vignette shows.

Wade was a capable, intelligent young man who had graduated at the top of his class from a very prestigious university. He was now in an executive training program of a major corporation. There was no doubt that if he completed the program he would rise to the top of the executive ladder. Yet he felt that life had lost its meaning and that he needed to be in some other career than business. He wavered between wanting to be a priest or a lawyer, careers seemingly at opposite ends of the spectrum in terms of material rewards. This is the point where his search for glory makes its appearance. It seems that both his parents venerated material success. They were opting for law as a choice, associating it with obtaining wealth. Wade's conflict was his need to complete the glory desired by his parents versus his need to fight against it. The parents' strong veneration of material success and the patient's identification with their values was blinding him to what his real self wanted. His self-ruminations were paralyzing him with painful indecision.

I asked him to clarify further what he meant in terms of the conflict between spirituality (the priesthood) and material success (a lawyer). The way Wade had stated the conflict appeared nebulous and, partly for my sake and his, I wanted him to clarify his thinking. Was it possible to amalgamate the two? What was in back of the blurring of the conflict? How did the conflict connect with his parents' desires? I wanted more details about the battle as I conceived it between the desire to satisfy his real self and the idealized self, which was a construction of both him and his parents.

Wade responded earnestly to the questions and my probing. What emerged from his real, authentic self was the desire to make some notable contribution to his parents' country of origin, a third-world country, in a "cause" greater than himself. But this "cause" was tarnished because in his mind it brought him closer to his enveloping parents. He had to progress in treatment to the point where his real self felt sturdy enough to embrace his true desire (i.e., working for an altruistic, humanistic cause) and know that he would not lose his self to his parents in the process.

As we have seen from the preceding vignettes, as a consequence of the conflicts between solutions, pride, self-hate, "shoulds," self-idealization, and the pursuit of glory, the patient struggles to "glue" himself together. The center of his being appears not to be there for him or threatens to weaken, causing panic or terror. To prevent this catastrophic event from occurring, the character disorder develops the idealized image. Once the idealized image is in place, he now has a glorious mission, a promising future, and a formidable project. He also has a spurious sense of momentary self-confidence. The idealized self acts like a pathological magnet, drawing to itself ersatz self-confidence and purpose.

Each of the neurotic solutions, when coupled with the idealized image, becomes transformed or reframed. Agreeableness becomes worthiness; anger becomes assertion; love becomes purity. But the idealized image grows like a cancer and in time conquers the character disorder's entire self (Horney, 1950a, p. 22). The patient may be completely unaware of this insidious process because of his alienation from his real self. The idealized image also stimulates a driven need for perfection, ambition, and glory. Aspirations become unrealistic. The goals take varied forms: power, massive wealth, gambling success; prestige, admiration (Horney).

Another significant element associated with the pursuit of glory is vindictiveness. The goal is to cause others to be envious of one's attainments, to shame them and in general cause them to be humiliated and defeated. The character disorder's need for a vindictive triumph is mainly directed toward those individuals perceived by him to have thwarted, opposed, or hurt him in the past. One patient told me jokingly that he chiefly bought a lottery ticket so that he could savor the delectable thought of denying some of his winnings to various people he hated and believed had hurt him in his career.

The frantic ambition of the character disorder masks the search for glory and vindictiveness. To the patient it is perfectly natural to sacrifice the basic needs of his family in the compulsive pursuit of success. He feels unable to modulate his zeal and rationalizes his laser-like career devotion, saying to his spouse, "When I make my first million I'll ease up and really be there for you and the kids." In my experience it seldom happens, because the absolute safety that the character disorder desires is never obtained.

The desire for glory reveals itself in many ways, chiefly the compulsive pressure to be the center of intelligence, that is, the most logical, the most knowledgeable, the most creative, the worthiest, the healthiest, the center of attention.

The following vignette illustrates how idealized glory perpetuates frustration in career choice and self-hate.

Gavin looked depressed. Asked what was going on, he told me that he had been at a party with some of his very wealthy friends, considerably more wealthy than he was. They had talked about their huge boats, private planes, and numerous residences in various parts of the country. He felt poor and ashamed by comparison even though he had inherited many millions from his father. His friends, though, had made their vast fortunes on their own, intensifying the patient's feeling that he was an inadequate fraud. He was continuing to struggle unsuccessfully during therapy to create an income, to earn money through his own efforts. What was paralyzing his efforts was a powerful drive to remain "safe" and only dependent on his inheritance. He was fearful of risking his finances invested in various stocks, in part due to a lack of confidence in his own judgment. His father had been unusually successful in his investment tactics but he had had an ambivalent desire to impart his invaluable skill to the patient before he died.

In spite of Gavin's statement that he had approached his father many times, eager to absorb the man's obviously astute stock market investment expertise, he revealed in therapy a self-defeating entitlement to be the possessor of his father's knowledge without any expenditure of energy on his part. He and I were able to piece together his probable, past self-destructive interaction that may have annoyed his father.

His father would begin to teach him, then abruptly and irritably dismiss him. The patient claimed to never know why this happened. While we were attempting to understand the "mystery" of his father's dismissal of him, Gavin was going for many job interviews but was not being hired. Investigation of the details of his behavior during the interviews revealed that he would inevitably insert, during an exchange with the prospective employer, that he really didn't need the money. The industry that he was looking to break into thrived on "lean and hungry" workers and Gavin was coming across as passive, self-satisfied, and self-effacing. His father had been in the same industry that Gavin aspired to but his father had been a very successful "shark," a savvy competitor with the very qualities that the patient lacked. In therapy, Gavin learned that he was trying to compete with his father in his search for glory and that he would stand a better chance of gaining a measure of happiness if he utilized his own very different, good assets. His pursuit of glory was only increasing his self-hate and self-frustration.

Horney (1950a, p. 33) addressed the role of imagination or daydreams fueling the search for glory. She (Horney, p. 31) stated that we are always imaging fictitious scenarios in the process of self-idealization. Horney (p. 31) declared "No matter how much a person prides himself on being realistic, no matter how realistic indeed his march toward success, triumph, perfection, his imagination accompanies him and makes him mistake a mirage for the real thing." When fantasy crowds out reality, we suffer psychosis. By the way, there is no adequate definition of reality. The one I have found most useful is when the patient really knows what matters or what should be his priority. I have found that character disorders distort reality in terms of the preceding definition.

THE ROLE OF FANTASY

All actions and verbalizations are creatively first begun with fantasy. Horney (1950a) recognizes that fantasy initiates and builds the idealized image. In the process of constructing the idealized image, reality is played with, altered, and falsified. Thus a mere stated intention, a mechanical "I'm sorry," becomes authentic and complete to the character disorder, and the action substantiating the contrition does not have to be initiated. It also is a fantasy at work when the ephemeral thought of greatness, the parroting of morality and values, ensures their existence. In the mind of the individual suffering from character pathology no further action need be taken.

Horney (1950a, p. 35) compares the character disorder to Goethe's Faust, who desired to be omnipotent and omniscient. His desire was granted by the devil when Faust agreed to the devil's pact. Of course, there were strings attached to the pact, leading to the loss of Faust's soul. Loss of pieces of reality always have pernicious consequences for the character disorder, ranging from a slight emotional and/or physical disability to more serious and profound disruptions of the self.

The character disorder, caught in the grip of his idealized image, will not accept or wish to see immovable, realistic limitations to his claims or the attainment of his specific glory. He may, according to Horney (1950a, p. 36), be repelled by the real and the obvious. Limitations of time and energy do not apply to him. The idea of his ultimate death is fearfully avoided. Obvious cause and effect relationships are negated, such as, "If you eat excessively and do not exercise, you are not supposed to gain weight."

Horney (1950a, p. 38) again asserts a basic premise of her theory and therapeutic technique. It is her recognition that the real self strives toward self-realization. By contrast, the pursuit of glory, an outcome of the action of the idealized self, opposes the real self's determination to grow. The real self stands for spontaneity, recognizing limitations, development, and presence. On the other hand, the pursuit of glory, in thrall to the idealized image, exemplifies a glorious accomplishment, rejecting limits, pretending and living mainly in the imagination.

The following vignette dealing with the patient, Ellen, is an example of how the idealized image creates a false, pathological sense of significance and a neurotic solution of self-effacement and doubt. The pursuit of glory is also enforced.

Ellen settled into the chair and I waited for her opening remark, as I usually do with all my patients. She leaned forward and asked, "Do you have a pencil and paper?" Her question naturally evoked curiosity as to why she wanted these items, but I silently kept my thought to myself and complied. She bent over the table between us and swiftly drew a circle and arrows pointing to this circle. "You see, this circle is me and my anxiety" and she drew a wavy line on the circle's line. "These arrows are all the people and other things causing me tension." She began labeling them. "This is my husband. My brother is here. Here is my father. That one is my mother. Here is my male friend and this one is my best girlfriend. This diagram is to show you just where I am now in the best way I know how." I thanked her and asked how each person intruding upon her caused and increased her anxiety.

"My husband wants me to make up my mind and stay in the marriage. My stepson from my husband's previous marriage feels very close to me and loves me. He would be just devastated if I divorced his father. My father would be happy if I left my husband. My mother would throw a party if I said "Goodbye" to my husband. She hates him. My brother feels the same way as my mother. My male friend feels I ought to leave my husband. My girlfriend is ambivalent. She likes my husband in one sense, probably because by staying with him I remain geographically close to her and she can get to me easily with her problems."

Ellen experienced them all pushing on her, almost all pretty much certain of the correctness of their position in urging her to give up on her marriage. It was only Ellen who was uncertain about what to do. When her husband gave vent to paranoid accusations about her possibly cheating on him, Ellen would flee their apartment to another apartment she kept as a place of refuge. There, she would be certain she needed to leave her husband. Her husband would then call, appeal to her to come back, and her resolve would melt. And so it went back and forth with all the people and the arrows surrounding her drawn circle awaiting her ultimate decision.

I understood from Ellen's history that her mother and father had ended their marriage when the patient was 9 years old. They continued to live under the same roof for another 10 years. Both she and her brother were confused by this marital arrangement. She witnessed the father's frequent rages (somewhat like her husband's) and her mother's numbness (akin to Ellen's experience when her husband ranted and raved against her during a quarrel).

In therapy she and I came to see that her marriage recapitulated her parents' ruptured marriage. But how did the pursuit of glory enter into this melange? The answer was the circle, representing Ellen. Despite the stress of so many people wanting her to finally decide what to do about her marriage and move on, what counted most was that she had their undivided attention. That's what she wanted and needed. She remembered that as a child she was forgotten by both her parents as they were going at each other. Her glory now was to have every significant person in her life wait on her. She had the power now (the power of the seemingly powerless) that she never had as a child, and she was undoubtedly savoring it. Every time her family or friends would begin to talk about their worries, Ellen would adroitly pull them back to her plight. She would do it with agitated displays of depression and suicidal attempts. Her family thought it strange that she remained with her husband given his flagrant, inappropriate, rageful acting out. Her decision to remain with her husband replicated her parents' separation where they had remained with each other for a long time despite being divorced for all intents and purposes. They had lived under the same roof and continually quarreled. Ellen was able to inflate her idealized image by emphasizing her importance to her husband, the stepson, her family, and two friends. At first it appeared that the patient's idealized image was not inspiring self-confidence; a necessary component of the search for glory was lacking. A closer examination revealed that she was confident about never failing to bring those individuals closer to her if they drifted away from her marital quandary.

The next vignette of the patient, Keith, illustrates the emphasis an individual with an idealized image often places on appearance rather than being.

Keith entered therapy complaining of depression and an increasingly greater expansion of disappointment in the way his career was progressing. My first impression of the patient was that of a natty appearance. He was very dapper, wearing a gray suit and pink tie, and his hair was carefully combed back. He looked every inch the successful lawyer. Speaking about himself there was a clear pattern of an emphasis on appearance. He had selected his wife because of her exotic look. He and his wife would occasionally dress alike to attract the attention of a dinner crowd at a restaurant or participants at a cocktail party. As soon as he could afford it, he purchased a "drop dead" house in a very exclusive area to impress his friends and family. He would search car magazines to discover what auto would give him the greatest prestige.

Everything he did was done with an eye to appearance. He had to associate with people of status and wealth. He had to feel that the sub-specialty of law he practiced was special and elitist. His office wall was covered with diplomas, certificates, plaques, and testimonials attesting to his professional competence and fame.

When he first entered his profession, he imagined that he ultimately would be at a point where his colleagues would eagerly beat a path to his door. They would recognize his superior legal mind and want to appoint him to their law school faculty. It did not happen and he furiously blamed the influx of women who displaced very capable male professionals like himself.

Keith seemed to be a detached individual who appeared to have a distant relationship with his wife and children. He could be very critical and perfectionistic. Most of the time he felt as if he knew more than most of the people he met. He would inevitably slip into a conversation statements about where he lived and the kind of car he drove. He did not seem to be really interested in the other person's feelings or concerns except if he could exploit them in some way.

Given his idealized image of smugness, belief in his omniscience, and superior knowledge, he expected to be in a position of power with concomitant fame. He had convinced himself before he embarked on his career that his imagined success was an actuality. Now as we unpacked the various elements of his idealized image and its vision of glory, he was becoming more aware that it was only a veneer, not an actuality. He went through a mourning period as he painfully had to let go of his dream of glory.

At this point I would like to compare and contrast a paper, "The Golden Fantasy: A Regressive Reaction to Separation Anxiety" (Smith, 1977), with Horney's (1950a) concept, "The Search for Glory," because I see it in many ways as an extension of Horney's seminal thinking. As is typical of Freudian journals, Horney (pp. 31–36) is not cited as a significant contributor to Smith's excellent paper, but her thinking (i.e., her linking imagination to glorious fantasies) is apparent in his discussion.

Smith (1977) emphasizes the importance of fantasy in psychoanalytic treatment. I would add that it is, of course, significant in psychotherapy as well. The therapist's goal is to uncover fantasies that determine behavior. The unconscious fantasies embody wishes and important historical data. Horney would certainly agree with Smith that the exploration of the patient's imagination is vital toward further progress in therapy. The "Golden Fantasy" for Smith (p. 311) means *"the wish to have all one's needs met in a relationship hallowed by perfection."* Horney would add that the "Golden Fantasy" is probably a variation of her concept, the search for glory, encountered in every character disorder. She would argue that the "Golden Fantasy" includes a person out for perfection in thinking, career, wealth, health, etc. Horney no doubt would agree with Smith that passivity or self-effacement plays a key role in contributing to the production of the fantasy.

Horney (1950a) saw the idealized image as linked to the pursuit of glory and as a means of holding the self together. Smith too sees the role of the "Golden Fantasy" as a prime source of comfort and bestower of meaning. As Smith (1977, p. 311) states, "It is as if the fantasy provided a self definition: without it there is no existence and the world becomes a place without hope." Although Smith asserts that the "Golden Fantasy" first appears within the transference, I have seen it revealed in the patient's relationships with others, such as the patient who exhibits a narcissistic entitlement, expecting a husband to meet all of her needs and have none of his own in the marriage. I see claims, "shoulds," and the search for glory as excellent pointers to the existence of the "Golden Fantasy." Like Smith's "Golden Fantasy" concept, Horney views the search for glory in a sense as an intrinsic aspect in all character disorder pathology. Smith introduces developmental issues specifically responsible for the production of the "Golden Fantasy." He sees it as the experience of the loss of the mother during the separation-individuation stage (Mahler, Pine, & Bergman, 1975). The loss can be due to the mother's narcissism, a new baby, or any physical separation engendering abandonment feelings in the patient. The effects of the loss are significant because it may come shortly after Mahler's symbiotic phases where supposedly Mommy and I are one.

The "Golden Fantasy" is the patient's attempts to reclaim the wonderful passive sense of oneness with a life-giving other. Horney's clinical observation of the character pathology and the search for glory seem to point to the regressive urge to recapture blissful dependency.

Smith (1977, p. 314) perceives the fantasy as intensifying resistance and the resolving of a formidable blockage pivotal to the success of therapy. A sign of the "Golden Fantasy" resistance is acting out (e.g., possibly an affair). In effect the patient says, "I can do without you. There are others who will be able to satisfy my fantasy." If this behavior happened while a patient was engaged in therapy, Horney would probably see the acting-out as the patient's vindictiveness toward the therapist for not improving the effectiveness of the pursuit of glory.

Donna, a patient previously mentioned, is an example of acting out the "Golden Fantasy." She longed for the man she had had an affair with many years ago. This affair took on in her imagination the personification of everything she had ever desired in an intimate relationship or marriage. She kept toying with the idea of contacting him with the hope that he might leave his wife and she and he would go off into the sunset.

The following is another example of compulsive acting-out of the "Golden Fantasy" and/or the search for glory. The consequences were dire for both the patient and his family.

Norman had a wonderful job, a loving wife, and two children. But occasionally his wife criticized him for some of his adolescent behavior. Her reproof was accompanied by her sexual withdrawal. This deeply rankled him. Norman, who was proud of his persuasive verbal skills and employed them in his acting-out, would randomly telephone women whom he'd never met and attempt to persuade them to meet him at a nearby hotel. His verbal ability and manipulative capability was so superior that it sometimes worked. He was actually able at times to convince a woman to meet him at a nearby motel to consummate their mutual sexual desires. When he succeeded in persuading a woman, a total stranger, he would momentarily feel that his pursuit of glory was validated; it epitomized the power of his persuasive facility. But his compulsive sexual need mixed with glory-seeking would not let him rest. He was finally apprehended by the police and charged with making obscene phone calls. His whole world, his profession, his family, fell apart.

I had tried many times in sessions to ground Norman in the dire consequences of his compulsion, but he was completely caught up in the strong current of sexual glory-gratification. Unlike his wife, each of the women he had called had at that moment of success become the perfect woman who would fulfill his every emotional and sexual wish.

Smith (1977) brings out another repercussion of the "Golden Fantasy" that Horney does not, to my mind, sufficiently elaborate. He finds certain patients guilt-ridden and so ashamed of the content of their fantasy that they substitute rejection of the therapist instead of rejection of the fantasy. They expect the therapist to be judgmental and to find them repugnant. Horney (1950a) however, does write about the process of externalization, where the patient projects disowned specific wishes and needs, and sees them as belonging to the therapist. Externalization would then explain the patient's heightened hostility and criticality toward the therapist.

According to Smith (1977), drawing closer to the therapist and endowing him as the main satisfier in the fantasy may trigger the frightening horror of suffocation or being swallowed up. Horney (1950a) handles that resistance in her discussion of the morbidly dependent character disorder and other neurotic solutions.

Both Smith and Horney recognize that authentically committing oneself to therapy means the painful relinquishment of a pleasurable, glorious fantasy as an essential step toward gaining a realistic measure of happiness.

PRIDE

Attempting to attain self-esteem, the character disorder, no matter what the solution, fails to arrive at his ambitious goal. No matter how much he redoubles his efforts, no matter how much he gives vent to perfectionistic strivings, to the "Golden Fantasy," the glory continues to elude him. How to replace the blow to his self-esteem when he fails to attain glory? The answer is neurotic pride linked to the idealized image. With neurotic pride the character disorder can depart from reality and believe he has convincing merits, thereby restoring his self-esteem.

Healthy pride, according to Horney (1950a, pp. 88–109), is having self-authored values, taking responsibility for one's self, having realistic knowledge of one's capabilities, liabilities, and potential, expressing genuine feelings directly, and having mature interpersonal relationships.

It is proper to be proud of extraordinary accomplishments and to admire them. This sensible pride is characterized by a modest dignity and self-worth.

The unhealthy pride of the character disorder is tinsel grounded on a haughty, idealized image. In our society, neurotic pride may emphasize the compensatory pursuit of prestige, such as brand name watches, clothes, status cars, association with the "beautiful" people and the ultra-wealthy, or boasting about a family member's academic or career attainments.

The character disorder may attach pride to his high intellect, supposed deep feelings, fair judgment, excellent reasoning, and determined ambition. These qualities are enveloped in clouds of glory. Usually, what the character disorder is most proud of in himself exists only in his imagination. He slights or injures who he really is. His narcissistic self-assessment, helped by his alienation from himself, becomes the basis of claims and "shoulds." What counts now is to effectively assert the claims and "shoulds" (e.g., to manipulate, cheat, control, avoid responsibility for one's actions, as in the case of the patients, Tyrone or Betty, who were overdependent subtly or openly demanding and selfish).

A character disorder may be proud of his suffering, supposed humility, cynicism, bargaining skills, vindictiveness, or risk-taking.

The next vignette conveys a patient's pride in his willingness to enter into clearly life-threatening situations.

The patient, Jerry, 70 years old, was proud of his past treks into scary areas. He had once hitchhiked by himself through an African nation in the throes of civil war where fatal attacks were not uncommon. Another time, he went into a Rio De Janeiro barrio at night, despite being warned by the police stationed on the periphery that he was risking his life and that they, heavily armed and in groups of four, would not dare to go through the streets.

When the patient arrived I noticed that he was perspiring. Instead of answering my question about why he was perspiring he volunteered that he was having trouble seeing. I knew that he had had cataract surgery for both eyes but one eye was still giving him a great deal of trouble, limiting his vision. I recalled that he prided himself on biking through New York City traffic, a perilous undertaking even for those with excellent vision and supreme reflexes. Given the magnitude of his unhealthy pride, I could have anticipated his response to my next question: "Are you still riding your bike?" I was hoping that he would say "Are you crazy?" That was not to be. He smiled and said, "Yes, I am and I don't have any accidents." I continued, "You seem proud that you risk your life, considering your very impaired vision and other physical conditions." He retorted, "I like taking risks. Besides, how am I to get around New York?" Ironically, despite seeming to court obvious physical dangers, Jerry was unable to take other, emotional risks, so I confronted him with this. "I would like you to consider why you make placing yourself in a potentially dangerous situation a virtue, a badge of courage, yet when it comes to going to a dance where you could possibly meet a woman, you back away and say 'I don't want to take a chance because they probably are all unattractive.'" I was presenting him with the existing, glaring contradiction between his supposed courage in the face of a real threat to life and limb and his anxiety about being rejected if he risked reaching out to a woman. He had filled previous sessions with numerous complaints about his painful loneliness and heartfelt desire to have a female companion. Jerry, in the grip of self-hate, had poor self-esteem. He could only respond to a woman's overtures if she was very aggressive at their first meeting and made clear to him that she desired him. Her signals of approval of him had to be loud and unambiguous.

The following dialogue between myself and a patient conveys her embrace of prestige and social status and the consequent spurious inflation by the idealized image of ersatz self-worth.

Betty, a patient previously mentioned (the one proud of her beautiful garden and desiring her son to be married in it), was talking to me about her future daughter-in-law. She opined, "I come from a refined family. My daughter-in-law does not." I asked, "Does she know how you feel about her family?" "I keep it hidden." I offered an intervention at this point, "Maybe she knows anyway about your pride in your family and your feeling that it is better than hers, and it makes her angry. You did say that she is often angry with you." I suggested the preceding view based on the patient's frequent, proud allusions to the elevated social status of her parents. It seemed to me likely that Betty could not refrain from boasting pridefully before anyone, especially her future daughter-in-law, and savoring her superiority. I was attempting to help the patient increase her awareness of her character deformation, her competitive, sneering devaluation of her daughter-in-law specifically and of people in general.

The following vignette is an example of how pride in virtue and saintliness can paper over a need to control, manipulate, and make others feel uncomfortable through guilt-producing pestering.

Henry took great pride in his willingness to give to charities and to offer a helping hand to those "poor souls" who through cruel fate suffered physical limitations or were barely clinging to life. This trait would certainly be termed very admirable if it were not for one additional characteristic. He wanted, wished, claimed, and felt compulsively entitled to relentlessly pressure his friends to be as charitable and giving to the needy as he was. His friends would politely decline and wish him well with his project. But Henry would not retreat. He would approach them again, this time employing guilt-producing comments, such as "Don't you think you are being selfish?" and "Look at me, I have little time and energy yet I give of myself." His wife and many of his friends were alienated by Henry's stubborn pressures.

When I presented him with the deleterious consequences of his inappropriate manipulation, his jaw would be set firmly and he would say determinedly "I don't care. I know that I'm right and if I find one person who agrees with me that will prove I'm right." Henry's massive pride in his virtue had impaired his normally decent intelligence, so much so that his nonacceptance of another's right to feel differently than he did just did not count.

Once pride is detected in any one sector, Horney (1950a) suggests that the therapist look for the connections pride has to many facets in a character disorder's makeup. In the case of Henry, for example, pride was attached to egocentricity, the frustration of others, stubbornness, domination, insensitivity, and obsessiveness. He also demanded that he should be pampered wherever he went.

The therapist needs to become aware of all the prides of a patient. The patient will fight "tooth and nail" to preserve any character trait that is invested with pride. He may feel that his pride plus his trait gives him an edge, be it the smug belief in his superior intelligence or intuition, his virtue or assertiveness.

Horney (1950a, p. 95) postulates that pride contributes to the patient's vulnerability. She notes that there are two main consequences of hurt pride. These are shame and/or humiliation. She differentiates the two, seeing shame as a feeling we put on ourselves when we think that we have done something wrong, while humiliation is our conviction that others are censoring us. In any case she determines that as therapists we need to obtain details about a particular pride; that is, under what circumstances it occurs and how it is expressed.

Here is an example of the importance of distinguishing between shame and humiliation, depicted in the interaction between myself and a patient.

> THERAPIST: *If your son could enter an occupation that he enjoys and can do well that would be growth.*
>
> PATIENT: *Not if he wants to be a carpenter. My family consists only of professionals. They would look down on him.*
>
> THERAPIST: *You sound as if you would feel humiliated.*
>
> PATIENT: *You bet!*

The patient rigidly adheres to a "should," that of believing that only the status of a professional career is correct for his son. Given the ongoing conflict between him and his son, one would expect that he would welcome any career choice that his son would make that would bring his son a gratifying identity and the satisfaction of honest competence. Priorities and reality become impaired when pride enters the arena, as this father's reaction clearly shows.

Each type of character disorder, according to Horney (1950a), reacts differently to injured pride. The aggressive expansive character disorder will brush off any threat to their pride. They will not feel shame for they are convinced that they are perfect. They will become hostile to anyone who questions whatever their pride covers up in themselves.

Self-effacing character disorders will feel some humiliation if their pride is attacked but shame will be more intense.

If the patient is self-righteous, shame will be put down and pride preserved.

The arrogant, grandiose character disorder can not admit that he has been hurt or has made a mistake, as the following vignette shows. The patient is Tyrone, the unscrupulous businessman whom we have met before.

> THERAPIST: *Tyrone, you don't seem to feel shame or humiliation no matter what you do.*
>
> PATIENT: *Why should I? I just put my foot over the boundary of the law. When they slap my hand I step back. So now I'll try something else.*

Horney (1950a, p. 98) observes that hurt pride can take many diverse forms, such as shame, a vague discomfort, guilt, vindictive anger, irritability, or rage. She (Horney, p. 99) points out that hurt pride can be discerned when it has elements of disdain, contempt, or vindictiveness.

A patient may turn against herself if she feels that she can no longer be proud of a character trait, in this case letting herself down in terms of independence, as the following vignette demonstrates.

> *The patient had attempted suicide and I was seeking to find out what was the precipitating cause.*
>
> PATIENT: *I went into the bathroom and cut my arm.*
>
> THERAPIST: *That was after you said you were not going with your husband to his parents.*
>
> PATIENT: *That's right.*
>
> THERAPIST: *Could there be a connection between your anxiety and him leaving you?*
>
> PATIENT: *I thought it would not bother me. I could be okay alone.*
>
> THERAPIST: *You became anxious.*
>
> PATIENT: *Yes. I have always been proud of the fact that he couldn't threaten me by going off. I wouldn't collapse if he left. Instead I felt like my whole world was coming apart. I felt mad at myself for being such a baby.*

The patient's injured pride took the form of a violent, suicidal act. Unrealistic, demanding "shoulds," as represented by the preceding vignette of the patient believing that she should never feel any anxiety, render a character disorder vulnerable and susceptible to injured pride. Anticipatory fears also play a role in impairing pride. Basically the character disorder is beset by two contradictory elements: pride and self-disdain, placing him in a constant state of anxiety.

Horney (1950a, p. 103) offers some insight into vindictiveness in terms of pride. Retaliation may be a vehicle to repair impaired pride. But the success of the vindictiveness has to be much greater than the offense in order to satisfy the patient and completely restore his damaged pride to his satisfaction. Recall the patient, Bob, who unrelentingly punished his aunt for more than a decade for not inviting him to her daughter's wedding.

There are other areas of the character disorder's life that are affected badly by damaged pride. Losing interest in one's profession, hobby, or any situation, for example, may be the result of injured pride. The patient may feel he would rather give up an activity than suffer failure. Existing perfectionistic standards almost ensure failure. Relationships, according to Horney (1950a, p. 105), may be given up as the character disorder senses dimly that the other person has failed him in some way or that he, himself, has disappointed his friend or marital partner. Pride and shame then prevent him from admitting it.

Attempts to restore injured pride can take many forms, including denial, forgetting, humor, objectivity, minimizing, reinterpretation so that the other is blamed, or a mechanical "I'm sorry." The bottom line in all these ersatz efforts to revive damaged pride is the avoidance of responsibility and the hiding of one's flaws.

In essence, the character disorder seeks safety and may avoid risk as a means of eluding possible hurt pride. The result may be restrictions in certain areas of one's life: alibis, a taboo on emotional risk taking or on entering into new, enriching life experiences. Horney (1950a, p. 129) concludes that all the circumstances of pride are the natural consequences of the pursuit of glory. The idealized image sets up unrealizable standards of performance in the shape of "shoulds" and demanding, assertive, prideful claims. Self-hate then inevitably mingles with injured pride.

7 The Initial Interview

When discussing the initial interview it is worthwhile to refer to Irvin Yalom (2002), who best expresses Horney's fundamental psychotherapeutic standpoint applicable to the first meeting and subsequent sessions with the patient. He (Yalom, p. 1) writes,

> When I was finding my way as a young psychotherapy student the most useful book I read was Karen Horney's *Neurosis and Human Growth*. And the single most useful concept in that book was the notion that the human being has an in-built propensity toward self-regulation. If obstacles are removed, Horney believed, the individual will develop into a mature, complete adult, just as an acorn will develop into an oak tree.

I have discussed hopelessness and the vital role hope plays in the success of treatment. One necessary goal of the initial session is to begin the process of instilling hope in the patient that he can change his life for a better existence.

THE ROLE OF HOPE

The expectation that hope could exist more powerfully in therapy was heightened by Horney's challenge to Freudians that development does not depend on immutable instinctive forces.

On the other hand she held cultural factors to be determinants of the personality, a supposition that opens a door of hope to possibilities for external action and that places current conflicts in the center of therapeutic action, while giving less importance to the conflicts of infancy (Manrique, 1984, pp. 301–302).

By contrast to Freud, Horney did not emphasize the role of sexuality, nor did she view as accurate a lock-step progression of personality as presented by Freud. "The important thing, according to Karen Horney, is not the active and sexual need to love, but the need to be loved" (Manrique, 1984, p. 302).

Horney stressed the importance of the individual's need for security and avoidance of fear. She emphasized that fear is not inborn but caused by a lack of acceptance by significant others.

Given all of Horney's basic modifications of Freud's seminal ideas, we have a much more malleable, less firm configuration than that defined by Freudian psychoanalysis. Horney asserted in her final, main summation of her ideas that an individual also has the capacity to become a reasonable person. She maintained that an individual can change and that he can evolve during his entire lifetime.

The factor of hope was intrinsic in Horney's work. It is absolutely mandatory for a positive therapeutic outcome. Horney emphasized that the patient must struggle against his illness. Illness was a failure of hope. Horney believed that this lack of hope could be apparent within the first session. She also knew that the patient must assume some responsibility for maintaining hope.

The therapist, like the patient, must also have hope with regard to his own continued growth as a person in addition to having hope abbout the patient positively changing. The patient can invariably sense when the therapist has lost heart. Hopelessness is poisoning and Horney recognized that many of her colleagues have been overcome by despair at not being able to help a patient but did not think of it as a quandary (Horney, 1950a, p. 181).

The main goal of the therapist in the initial session is to establish as quickly as possible a space that the patient will recognize as a zone of safety. Once that is done, the patient may feel comfortable enough to talk about whatever bothers him. During the first session the therapist also needs to instill the hope that therapy can alleviate his distress and offer him the tools to better understand himself so that he can more effectively deal with the many challenges that life brings.

Horney (1946a, p. 109) hypothesizes that at the beginning of therapy the patient is not really interested in himself as he truly is, despite the fact that he may believe he is. The therapist has the challenging task of helping the patient recognize that he is only or mainly interested in how he should be. The therapist must clarify the need to close the disparity between his idealized image and his real or true self.

Before going on to portray further what a Horneyan therapist keeps in mind as he conducts an initial interview, let us pause and briefly survey Horney's main theoretical ideas that were presented at length in the preceding chapters.

RECAPITUALIZATION

Karen Horney's (1950a) theory of neurosis, really character disorders, recognizes the influence of culture while viewing neurosis as a constellation of defenses designed to deal with basic anxiety. She concentrates on character structure rather than early childhood psychosexual experiences. Neurosis for Horney is essentially a character disorder, *a way of life in which the patient is compulsively driven by conflicting "shoulds," claims, idealized images, alienation from the self and implicit and/or explicit self-hate.*

Horney does not neglect the consequences of disturbed relationships in early childhood. She does delineate important neurotic elements in a family (e.g., being unloved, lack of empathy or safety, and hostility) that can cause children to feel anxious and insecure.

Central to Horney's definition of the neurosis are two core elements: basic anxiety and character deformation.

Horney defines basic anxiety as a belief that one is inferior, unimportant, abandoned, and constantly put in jeopardy. Consequently, the world is perceived as determined to deceive, wrong, abandon, assault, and begrudge.

The following is an example of one form, somatic, that basic anxiety can take.

Jesse experienced basic anxiety in the shape of periodic stomach aches and an anticipation of catastrophic doom. He wondered if he could ever pay his bills or successfully attain the necessary credentials or professional advancement. His early childhood was one of insecurity, with parents who physically and verbally abused him. They made no attempt to understand his capabilities, anxieties, and hopes. His character disorder embodied expansiveness and despair. He alternated between grandiose achievement fantasies and a continuing conviction that he could not avoid failure because of constraining bouts of passivity and inertia.

In *Neurosis and Human Growth* (1950a), Karen Horney's final major work, she grappled with an elusive concept, the real self. She saw the real self as a primary drive toward healthy growth and gratification, especially when liberated from the tentacles of neurosis. The real self, the possible self, is made up of talents and capabilities. In other words, the real self can be likened to a diamond surrounded by the idealized image, a false shell.

The idealized self is a compensation for feelings of weakness and inadequacy. The consequences flowing from the idealized self are either a conviction of arrogance and omnipotence or a despised, self-hating self. There is usually a compulsive striving to actualize the idealized self, called by Horney (1950a) the search for glory. Every pursuit of glory has its own constellation of solutions, prides, claims, and "shoulds." The idealized self is created when there is a need for a more comprehensive self-image. It is a neurotic solution to promote false self-confidence, "top-dog" beliefs, a false identity of power and significance; it essentially involves a process of self-glorification.

Horney (1950a) presents three major character structures or trends and their accompanying solutions. They are as follows:

1. Moving toward people and the solution of compliance and self-effacement.
2. Moving against people and the solution of aggression and expansiveness.
3. Moving away from people and the solution of detachment or freedom.

In my clinical experience, seldom does a patient display exclusively one solution; rather most patients indicate a mixture of all the major trends.

Patients who express complacency attempt to reduce basic anxiety by evoking an affectionate reaction. They value unselfishness.

Patients who show expansiveness strive for mastery. They hate helplessness. Their prominent traits are arrogance, vindictiveness, and perfectionism.

Patients who manifest detachment want freedom. They venerate self-sufficiency. They do not care about material success and usually feel they are better than anyone else. Basic anxiety is dealt with by moving away from people. They live a rather narrow existence, asking very little out of life to avoid being disappointed. Above all else, they do not want to be bothered. I just have one modification to add to Horney's clinical description. There are detached character disorders who very much strive for material success as a means of remaining strongly independent and detached from others.

Claims which are self-righteous entitlements and expectations are the character disorder's attempts to obtain satisfaction of narcissistic needs and wishes, such as, "I am entitled never to be criticized because I am a virtuous person," or "I claim receiving affection from you even as I say hurting things to you."

"Shoulds" are the constraining limits never to be questioned that the patient places on himself and others, such as, "I should be perfect or the other person should be always understanding."

Finally, there is the powerful alienation from the self that makes the work with the patient in treatment so difficult. He stumbles around in the dark, cut off from the formidable, unknown, dynamic elements within his deformed character structure. He is not the driver but the driven and does not know it; and worse yet, not only does he not know it but he may not want to know.

THE HORNEYAN ORIENTATION AND EXPLORATION DURING THE INITIAL SESSION

The Horneyan therapist maintains, according to Horney (1946a, p. 108), an accepting, tolerant attitude. He genuinely is not judgmental. The therapist believes that there are constructive forces within the patient and, if they can be resurrected then he will be able to correctly deal with his character disorder.

The patient may come to therapy with a feeling of superiority, whether it is in the area of love, sex, money, morality, intellect, or aesthetic sensibility. Recall the patient, Sid, who smugly asserted that he was superior in intellect to the therapist or could see reality more objectively than anyone else. The patient may expect therapy to make him perfect and believe his character disorder is not an essential part of him. He usually has determinedly persuaded himself that his idealized image is an asset. In addition, going to the dentist and therapy may be one and the same to him. So very often the therapist may sense that the patient assumes that he merely has to talk, that is to open his mouth, and the therapist, like the dentist, will do the rest.

As the patient tells his tale of woe in the initial session, the therapist has to keep in mind that some version of self-hate is always in the background and a sense of superiority is in the foreground, causing despair. The presence of self-effacement, for instance, may mask the self-torture and feeling of unworthiness. There may also be arrogant "shoulds" and feelings of humiliation (Horney, 1947, p. 128).

Prognosis is always better if self-hate and self-frustration conflict with fantastic claims that are out in the open. Their public display gives the therapist a chance to show the presence of self-hate and superiority; this can go a long way in fostering a solid working alliance. A good question to possibly ask of the patient, if the timing is correct, is "Perhaps there isn't even an answer to this yet . . . but what do you really want out of life or for yourself?" (Horney, 1949, p. 138).

Horney (1957b, p. 179) stresses that the therapist needs to find out what the patient wants from therapy and what he hopes to accomplish. We can not assume that we will be able to obtain complete diagnostic understanding. It is important to discover the constructive forces or elements in the patient, such as, capacity for self-reflection; tolerance for anxiety, frustration, and ambiguity and suspended judgment. We observe how the patient introduces himself. What is he interested in? Is the patient egocentric, hostile, easily distracted, rigid? We try to discern how much the patient is resigned, domineering, or dependent.

We determine the nature of the patient's pride, inhibitions, curiosity, honesty, and authenticity. Does the patient indicate suffering and what is his attitude toward his pain? Some degree of anxiety and/or depression can act as a powerful incentive to work on himself with the therapist as a partner.

Horney (1957b, p. 180) enjoins the therapist to assess how much of the real self has been damaged, such as, the degree of liveliness, openness. How much is the patient alienated from his real, true self? If it is possible, we try to determine moments of joy and upset in the patient's history. Again, if it is possible, we attempt to ascertain the patient's feelings regarding sex. If there is an absence of sex this is a bad prognostic sign. Is the patient tender, affectionate, or callous during sex? What does the patient expect in general from relationships? Not all the preceding questions suggested by Karen Horney need to be posed or answered in the first session but they should be kept in mind.

With regard to understanding the patient's interpersonal relations, Horney (1957b, p. 182) advises that we discern the number of warm, close relationships the patient has had and how giving he was in those connections. I would add as well, how capable is the patient of expressing gratitude? Particularly enlightening is knowing how the patient dealt with adverse situations or calamities in the past and currently. What are the possibilities of change? There may be existing real obstacles to positive change. The patient, for instance, may have a debilitating, deteriorating illness, have no significant person to offer support and/or warmth. Are there signs of a reliable work history? Are there any past psychotic episodes?

Horney (1957b, pp. 182–183) reminds us that the best source of understanding is how the patient comes across in the session. Is he confusing, excessively rigid, lucid, highly circumstantial, or obsessive? If the patient previously had therapy, did he feel abused? If so, this is a bad prognostic sign.

What do we say to the patient about our findings? Horney (1957b, p. 183) suggests the following:

> It may be difficult because . . . and then add that on the basis of constructive resources shown, such as energy, initiative, or honesty, we feel that something can be done. When the patient asks how long therapy will take, we can tell him it depends on him, on his energy, honesty and ability to reveal himself.

If we spot any signs of reluctance to undergo therapy, Horney (1957b) offers us her astute clinical observations as to how each character disorder will express their reservations. The self-effacing patient will show a great willingness to begin therapy but will not want anything for himself and will voice self-doubts about the possibility that it could benefit him. The expansive patient hates to admit faults, is rebellious and self-righteous. The resigned patient voices hopelessness, is sensitive to coercion, and wants freedom.

Passoni (1952, pp. 74–77), in the Horneyan *American Journal of Psychoanalysis*, presents some prognostic indicators that may occur during the initial sessions. A poor prognosis is indicated by "the existence of a rigid neurotic solution, such as a profound resignation" (Passoni, p. 76). Also, "Extensive externalization, cynicism, predominance of negativistic, hostile, contemptuous attitudes toward self and others, shallowness, self-rightousness, pride in neurotic suffering—all are very obstructive, almost prohibitive features" (Passoni, 1952, p. 76).

With regard to investigating the past, the important issue for Ivimey (1950a, pp. 38–47), an early colleague of Horney and contributor to her ideas regarding theory and therapy, is "What do the past memories mean for the patient now?" How the patient answers can shed light on the character disorder's possible need to use the past "to externalize, overemphasize suffering or blame others" (Ivimey, p. 42)."

Patients may overemphasize the past, block it out, or cloud it over. The patient may want to evoke obfuscating sympathy through the evocation of past memories of suffering. Horney in her first book, *The Neurotic Personality of Our Time* (1937, p. 141), notes that

> A second means of obtaining affection is by appealing to pity. The neurotic will bring his suffering and helplessness to the attention of others, the motto here being "You ought to love me because I suffer and am helpless." At the same time the suffering serves as justification for the right to make excessive demands.

The use of suffering reminds me of a self-revealing confession of a gifted therapist and instructor, Jules Nydes (personal communication, 1965), who shared with his class that his first therapist had completely fallen for his vivid, well-narrated tale of woe. Therapy had come to a complete standstill as the therapist listened to Nydes' dramatic, gripping suffering. He left his therapist and went to Theodor Reik, a colleague of Freud. In the first session Nydes once again began his report of his terrible suffering, when Reik intoned in a flat voice, "No rachmounis," a Yiddish expression meaning "No pity." Nydes informed us that this was a significant turning point in his therapy and he was able to move forward in his development. Reik intuitively halted Nydes' potentially potent blockage of therapy by letting him know in no uncertain terms that he was not going to be led down an enticing primrose path; he was not going to go down the same road to failure as the previous therapist.

The following vignettes depict initial sessions of three different patients treated by the author. All these first sessions reveal important prognostic indicators.

The first statement by Ivan was the announcement that I would find him most unusual and interesting, perhaps the most interesting patient I had ever met. He then followed up this self-promotion with a challenge tied to my name, "Are you really a 'Solomon'? Well you'd better be 'King Solomon' because you are going to need all your wisdom with me."

Given his loud, dramatic attempt to portray himself as special, it was relatively easy to infer that beneath his bravado and expansiveness there was a strong undercurrent of inadequacy and self-hate. He was trying too hard and too early to be competitive with me even as he was calling out to be rescued. His saying that I would need all the wisdom of King Solomon to deal with him meant to me that he was a very damaged individual unable to free his real self from his idealized self. It also meant that he wanted to be rescued by someone who had to have considerable skills to undertake this difficult challenge.

Ivan was a professional in a high-powered, aggressive occupation where his expansive facade served him well. He did not fare as well at home, where his wife did not appreciate his verbal abuse of her. It was at her urging that he entered therapy. His character disorder was long-term and the prognosis was guarded. Given his obvious pride in his dramatic, challenging front, the course of therapy would be a bumpy ride. Nonetheless, Ivan was likable and bluntly honest. He was lively and had maintained some positive, satisfying relationships with friends and colleagues. Thus, there were some good indicators predicting potential progress. As a consequence of therapy the patient was able to significantly control his provocative verbal abuse of his wife and reduce his pride in his combative, challenging posture. He and his wife were then able to work as an effective team dealing with family conflicts.

Horney (1950a, p. 349) observed that

> From dreams with constructive elements the patient can catch a glimpse even in the initial phase of analysis of a world operating within him which is peculiarly his own and which is more true to his feelings than the world of his illusions.

The following segment highlights the valuable role a patient's dream may play in elucidating a hopeful prognosis.

After her divorce, Tammy anticipated that she would create a new and better life for herself, such as new friends and an affable male companion. She had endured a marriage for many years where there was little love expressed toward her by her detached husband. She had even retired from her job after her divorce to clear time for a variety of educational and cultural experiences. Instead, she continued to live within narrow confines, not really reaching out for friendships nor possibly meeting a man with whom she might have a gratifying, intimate relationship.

In her dream Tammy conveys clearly the status of her real self. She dreamt that she now had a huge, spacious house with large rooms which flowed smoothly into each other. The house had two balconies. In the dream she speculated as to how she would decorate the balconies and wondered where the house was.

Both Tammy and I saw the house as a depiction of her hidden, subdued self; a potential for a wider, richer, more expansive existence. She had buried her *elan vitale* underneath a self-effacing trend and a timid idealized self desiring approval.

The patient, Sid, in the next vignette is an excellent example of someone who manifested an abundance of poor prognostic signs. Ultimately he terminated therapy, feeling quite satisfied with his character deformation.

Sid entered treatment initially because his wife pressured him to change. He would explode frequently into verbal rages or retreat into a silent, seething anger lasting for days on end. Toward his adolescent daughter, whom he claimed to love, he would deliver scathing criticism before her friends. He did not seem to mind when she suffered humiliation and embarrassment.

During the first session he pridefully told me that he was a perfectionist and felt quite superior in intellect to most people. I anticipated that he would soon feel superior to me and this proved to be the case. Every intervention in a session was met with facial scorn and extended silence. His only goal appeared to be delivering what he considered his wife's latest stupidity. He devalued his wife's wish for closeness and denied any desire of her for communication or resolution of a conflict between them as her attempt to control him. Both his wife's and daughter's suffering, caused by his stern, smug detachment and his reliable frustration of their legitimate wishes for understanding, were belittled by him as their weakness.

The abundant, bad prognostic signs were his callous indifference to his family's suffering, his self-righteousness, rigidity, closed mind to interpretations, alienation from his real self, and an unrelenting pride in all the preceding pathological traits. There was even a deep pride in being sadistic to both his family and others. At the same time that he ended therapy he announced to a startled wife that he had filed for divorce, the culmination of all the obstructive tactics in therapy, despite her continued entreaties to work on the marriage in therapy. He remained supremely and adamantly convinced that he was pursuing the correct course. Though Sid did not intend it consciously, it would appear that he was in the end offering his family relief from chronic, torturing suffering caused by him through his decision to divorce.

Martin, a prominent teacher and training analyst at the Horneyan American Institute for Psychoanalysis, offers in an informative and useful paper a number of suggestions to improve the effectiveness of the initial session. He (Martin, 1978, p. 105) stresses "that only what the patients say in their own words has real value." They have the answers to their own life and their own meaningful language and idiom. Every patient has his or her own rhythm and the therapist has to adapt to it. In the first interview, Martin makes it expressly understood that he wishes to be directed by whatever really matters to the patient. He suggests that they let their feelings and thoughts out in terms of what really matters. He emphasizes that they are in the therapy room to examine themselves and find out about themselves.

Once the patient opens up, Martin (1978, p. 106) in effect asks the patient to tell him what he sees, such as, "As you listen to what you have said what do you hear?" Horney (1987, pp. 99–100) refers to Martin's 1978 paper he presented on the value of emotional experience. While Horney thought his contribution was valuable, she wanted to include intellectual experiences and life experiences as well, which may expand the patient's understanding of himself.

If a patient mentions a feeling, it is useful, according to Martin (1978), to ask the patient how that feeling is manifested? He keeps bringing the patient back to his own words. He has found that this repeated ventilation of ideas leads to taking greater responsibility for their character disorder.

In a lecture on "The Analyst's Personal Equation," Horney (1957a, pp. 191–197) details counter-transference issues inherent in therapists with types of character disorders. She also reminds us that each character disorder possessed by a therapist may have certain merits as well as liabilities. The aggressive therapist, for example, "will not overlook the patient's hidden aggression, nor will he be afraid to tackle problems or to be direct in his approach" (Horney, pp. 194–195).

According to Horney (1957a, pp. 194–197), the compliant therapist has a compulsive need to be liked. He stresses the patient's assets and minimizes the patient's hostility. Compliant therapists are afraid of angering the patient. He avoids interpreting the idealized image and is too giving regarding fees and time. He is too sympathetic and wants to make the patient dependent on him. The compliant therapist tends to see therapy from the patient's point of view, too much so.

Horney (1957a, pp. 194–195) suggests that the aggressive therapist can be controlling, insensitive, and injure the patient's feelings. He may interpret too quickly, be dogmatic, and feel omniscient.

The narcissistic therapist, as Horney (1957a, p. 195) sees him, generalizes too much and types his patients. He feels impatient and/or hopeless if the patient rejects his interpretation. He believes that he is the only one who can help the patient.

The perfectionistic therapist, according to Horney (1957a, pp. 195–196), is tenacious and detail-oriented but does not see an overall meaning. He is didactic and controlling, relatively insensitive to the patient's feelings. He is controlled by his "shoulds." He may berate himself for not being the "perfect" therapist.

Horney (1957a, p. 196) states that the arrogant-vindictive therapist is not compassionate enough and is self-serving and self-righteous. He will foster dependency.

The detached or resigned therapist is seen by Horney (1957a, pp. 196–197) as too observing and not sufficiently feeling. He fears involvement so he does not stir up strong feelings. He can slip into hopelessness as he believes change seldom takes place. He wants quick results.

Horney (1957a, p. 197) suggests that the therapist monitor his counter-transference by attempting to get in touch with his feelings and connect them with the point in the session that triggered off the feeling. She advises that the therapist ask himself "Is this an appropriate feeling and how did it come about?" Horney (p. 197) concludes that "A constant effort to examine our reactions and even our associations and to relate them to what is going on in the patient is essential if we are to help the patient toward self-realization and to keep growing ourselves."

Wassell (1955), a Horneyan psychoanalyst extending Horney's characterizations regarding counter-transference, observes that in the initial phase of therapy, the patient either opposes, appeases, or avoids the therapist. He comments on possible counter-transference issues existing in the first session, such as the therapist believing he is a superior being (God). There may be pride in his intellect. He may give in to an idealization of the patient. The therapist may be too ambitious in trying to control and influence the patient, such as by being too sharp, too questioning. Another type of therapist functions overcautiously; he tries to placate and please the patient. Another type of therapist swamps the patient with a multitude of interpretations, not giving the patient an opportunity to gain insights on his own. Some therapists remain aloof as the patient thrashes about on his own.

Finally, in terms of diagnosis: What is the essential distinction between a neurosis and a character disorder? Miller (1977), a Horneyan analyst, attempts to answer this question. He states that although the character disorder says his anxiety is overwhelming him there is little sign that it is truly monumental. Any anxiety experienced, though, is badly handled.

8 Interpretation

In *Neurosis and Human Growth* (1950a), Horney's major work, she reports that a member of the audience during her lecture asked her when she was going to talk about psychotherapy. She answered that everything that she had said about character disorder, namely, claims, "shoulds," search for glory, self-hate, etc., had to do with therapy. Of course, she was right since, when the timing is right, the Horneyan therapist does present to the patient aspects of her ideas relevant to the patient's verbalizations. However, Horney did talk at length in her work about how the therapist was to communicate his interventions to the patient, and that is the substance of this chapter.

An interpretation or intervention is a tentative suggestion and is usually phrased in terms of the therapist's degree of certainty, such as, "Could it be that you might be unduly submissive to your wife?" versus "We definitely can see a pattern of excessive compliance in relation to your wife."

There are different types of interpreting. There is the uncovering intervention, which calls the patient's attention to what he does not know. Then there is the directive intervention, where the therapist calls the patient's attention to the presence of a problem or contradiction, an overreaction, a forgetting, or a blockage. Finally, there is the interpretation that may point out a constructive aspect of the patient's behavior.

Every time the therapist is contemplating whether to offer an interpretation he considers a number of elements. Will the intervention help? Will it impair or halt progress? Is the patient feeling abused? If he is, the therapist will hold back on an intervention, because inevitably a valid interpretation may threaten a treasured conviction such as a claim and increase anxiety in an already vulnerable individual.

Another consideration is the working alliance, and the therapist is advised to check and consider the strength or weakness of the alliance. Is it good or weakening, and if possible why? Interpretations should not be made at the end of the session. If little time is left in the session the patient will not be able to do anything with the intervention. The therapist needs to hear and understand how the patient processes the interpretation. Sometimes the patient's reaction to an offered understanding is more important than the content of the intervention. If the patient throws out a juicy "exit line" worthy of further exploration, we wait until next session no matter how tempting it can be to offer immediate feedback.

The following vignette illustrates a patient's "exit line," one that cries out for intervention. However, I had to restrain myself from interpreting until another session.

Paula, an attractive, light-skinned African American, whose light skin color played a very significant role throughout treatment, began therapy because she was depressed and had marital difficulties. She described her main conflict as shame versus affection. She was married to an African American who happened to be a much darker color than she was. Her shame rested on the knowledge that her husband was a very caring, loving man but his color distressed her. She mentioned that at times he appeared to her like a huge "gorilla," and as she reported this association she blushed and obviously felt very embarrassed.

As therapy continued, Paula reported a fantasy that began in childhood and still continued, that she was really "white" with all the "superiority" it suggested. She fancied that if she had married a white man, she could have passed for white and her life would have been a lot easier. She was also plagued by a repetitive dream that began when she married. In the dream she is soaking in a tub and feeling clean, nice, and relaxed when some shadowy figure pours a stream of feces into the tub. She would always awaken at this point, feeling horror and alarm.

She began to recognize in therapy that she was angry at her husband because his "primitive" color, she felt, dragged her down to a lower status. She saw that she provoked him in many subtle ways to release her anger and to punish him.

A gift from her husband which she brought to me gave me the opportunity to make what I considered an elegant, on-target interpretation. Paula's husband had given her a bas-relief of a woman, half black and half white. It seemed obvious to me that he was intuitively telling her that he knew about her main identity conflict and the idealized image she was pursuing. I delivered my understanding, thinking she was ready to be receptive, toward the end of the session, a mistake. Paula was silent and I thought she was thinking constructively about what I had just offered her. At the door she said, "So what does it all mean?" So much for my elegant intervention. Her "exit line" was for me a humbling event and I vowed from that point on never to offer an intervention toward the end of a session. I also promised myself that I needed to work more on judging the receptivity of a patient to a possible interpretation.

A basic rule of interpretation is to concentrate on what is the significant, obvious behavior, because there is less chance of the patient blocking when his behavior is close to the surface. Dealing with what is observable avoids having to grapple with all the many historical causes of behavior; consistently drawing the patient's attention to the surface character deformations supplies the intermediary links between the past and the present.

The following vignette illustrates a consistent, obvious, significant character trend linked to the patient's past family history.

Jesse came from a family where ridicule was the main disciplinary vehicle. Every time Jesse, who identified with his parents, sarcastically ridiculed his own children and wife or confessed that he felt transferentially ridiculed by me, we could then move more readily into a connection with his past childhood experiences. Eventually the patient was convinced, to his chagrin, that he was unfortunately carrying out what he had hated most as a child, the sadism of parental ridicule. This recognition sparked a strong determination to change.

There are surface attitudes that are most commonly interpreted. They are: (a) the patient's submission or submissiveness, (b) idealization of the therapist, causing the patient to want to please and appease, such as, the patient bringing in long dreams or fascinating childhood events, and (c) a surface attitude of detachment and aloofness.

While we interpret surface attitudes or the significant obvious, we need to keep in mind counter-transference, which can compel the therapist who wishes to be idealized or is detached to mishandle a patient's idealization or the patient's detached character trend.

Karen Horney stressed the interpretation of the surface because interpreting the most conspicuous neurotic trend of a patient gives the therapist the best chance of reaching the patient. The surface character trends, for example, may be excessive independence, a need to be loved, or a power drive.

The following vignette illustrates a patient's conflict between a desire to alleviate her suffering and a characterological need to control and slight the therapist. It is a good example of what I mean by the significant obvious; that is, the main trait of a character disorder that is easily discernible to both the therapist and the patient.

Linda would frequently do two things during a session. She would sneak a peek at her watch when I began to talk and would begin to make out a check at the end of the session. Her glance at her watch caused me to feel discounted and that I, in her mind, was wasting her time. At the same time, her check-writing style triggered anger in me at her controlling efforts to extend the session as she continued to talk about herself. These two annoying behaviors were certainly conspicuous in the session.

I decided to bring them to the patient's attention and interpreted their belittling and controlling implications. At first she minimized their characterological, neurotic consequences with "I merely glance at my watch because time is so brief and precious here and I just didn't have enough time to write a check ahead of time." This was followed by "I forgot." She finally accepted that she was being controlling and discounting, but it took a much longer time for her to realize to what extent she carried these two destructive traits into every part of her life.

THE PATIENT'S REACTION TO AN INTERPRETATION

Good things happen when a patient recognizes a character trend. It begins the process of restoring a sense of power over his behavior, raising a hope of change and a relief from suffering.

It is vital and useful to observe the tone with which the patient responds to an interpretation. The patient, for instance, may react to an interpretation with bravado, docility, defiance, arrogant superiority, or stony silence. We ask the patient to comment on his reaction. We also keep in mind the idea of why the patient reacts this way to an intervention. What does it have to do with what is happening in the session, with the therapist and the patient's interpersonal relationships?

According to Horney (1956b, pp. 212–213), in the therapeutic process there are many possible reactions to interpretations. The patient's pride may be hurt; he may feel humiliated, irritated; he may believe that the interpretation is unfair or see it as a condemnation of himself. Sometimes the patient is hostile because in his eyes he has shamefully exposed himself. Using externalization, the patient may feel the interpretation is an expression of the therapist's sadism. The patient may have silent reservations about the intervention or equate knowing with doing. The patient may not be grateful because the intervention inhibits his neurotic claims. On occasion the patient offers a pseudo-acceptance or, alienated from his feeling, he shows a form of dutiful acceptance. Horney (1956b, p. 214) also notes that

> Sometimes the patient seems interested and it appears that the interpretation has started something going, but soon, perhaps in the same hour, or the next, the patient's interest peters out. Such reactions occur in people who respond in the same way in life, with easily aroused enthusiasms which flag if love or success are not obtained quickly.

The following is an instance of an interpretation that was countered with wounded pride.

I had offered Carl the interpretation that he was angry at his wife but feeling more like a "man" because of her dependency upon him. He dismissed my intervention as not applicable to him. He then went on to explain and boast how a "man" does not complain and that he had once been a past commander of the Veterans of Foreign Wars. He informed me proudly that he was respected there as a leader because he never whined. My interpretation was dismissed because Carl saw it as casting aspersion on his manhood and as a distasteful definition of him as a whiner. Never mind that each session the patient complained bitterly about his wife's controlling dependency. He did not want to see it as whining at that moment. This time, the significant obvious was being rejected.

The following is an example of the same patient, Carl, his externalization of his self-hate, and his perception of my interpretation as a threat to a rigorously held claim.

Carl was furious with his son. He saw him as inadequate and worthless. I presented him with the possibility and understanding that he felt that same way about himself since he was retired now and was no longer a boss who gave orders to others. I speculated aloud that he may feel that he lost power and was becoming enfeebled. "No! Definitely not!," he replied. "It is my worthless son that I'm talking about."

He was reacting to my intervention as if it was a threat to his claim to be superior to his wimpy son, as he saw him. If he let my interpretation in he would be feeling self-hate. It was much more satisfying to hate his son.

INTERPRETING HOSTILITY

Horney (1936, p. 62) discusses at length how a patient may feel hostility toward a therapist after receiving a good interpretation, "as if the analyst, by seeing something they had not seen, is proved more intelligent, clear-sighted, or more articulate than the patient—as if the analyst had asserted his superiority over the patient." She continues by pointing out that the patient may express his hostility in subtle ways, such as wondering aloud whether he, the patient, could have said the same thing more elegantly. More directly, the patient may belittle the therapist or quite outrightly refuse to cooperate.

Horney refers to the competition inherent in our culture, furthering rivalry with the therapist in certain patients. "Their feeling toward life is that of a jockey in a race; they are dominated by the question, am I ahead? . . . These patients expect tremendous admiration and they have, in addition, fantastic expectations of their capacity for accomplishments" (Horney, 1936, p. 63).

Hostility in the patient may be engendered because of inordinate, unrealistic ambitions characterized as "No one but I shall be a good musician, read a good paper; no one but I shall be attractive, praised, or get attention and care when sick" (Horney, 1936, p. 63). Horney (pp. 63–64) mentions that hostility may take the form of extraordinary sensitivity to what the patient falsely perceives as the therapist's criticism of him. Even though the patient will benefit from a good interpretation, Horney finds, they may feel hostile; they are threatened that the therapist may in some ways know them better than they know themselves. Their pride in their self-sufficiency appears to them to be under attack. The patient may express antagonism toward the therapist because he feels humiliated, seeing the interpretation as exposing weakness.

> They feel humiliated, therefore, if one uncovers nothing more than the fact that they are in a dilemma, that they have certain anxieties, and that there are irrational elements in their expectations. They react as if they automatically translated the analyst's reference to "anxiety" into "cowardice," "sensitivity" into "effeminacy," etc. (Horney, p. 64).

For many patients "It has always hurt the patient to be dimly aware of flaws in his personality" (Horney, 1936, p. 64). This type of patient will feel veiled hostility or a reduction in his self-respect when he is reprimanded by the therapist.

Horney (1936, p. 65) entertains the possibility that the patient's ill will may be fueled by a more convoluted thinking but nonetheless a powerful dynamic constellation of feelings. The patient may fear benefiting from a good interpretation. Horney (p. 65) postulates that for the patient success is equated with maliciously triumphing over his conquered adversaries who will attack him if he successfully embraces the good interpretation. Therefore, the patient expresses anger toward the therapist, who is seen as an adversary prepared to attack him for his victory.

A number of Horneyan analysts have followed Horney's pioneering study of hostility and humiliation. Van Bark (1959, pp. 21–27), for instance, offers a useful direction in interpreting the patient's hostility. She finds it helpful to enlist the patient's enthusiasm for exploring the complexity of reactions that he or she may refer to as "mad," "blew my top," or "pissed" and to connect this feeling with the preceding and subsequent context, such as, "You say you blew your top when your son did so and so. Let's look more closely at your 'blowing your top.' It may be a lot more complex. It's usually more helpful to you if you try to understand it that way." Exploration of the concomitant defensive structure also helps in expanding the patient's appreciation of the nuances of his or her rage and aggression and—I would add—other aspects of his character structure.

Landman (1959), a Horneyan analyst, thinks that Horney's theory of neurosis explains hostility quite well and offers interpretative suggestions. She sees hostility as a method of defending the status quo of the neurotic defensive system. I would say hostility defends the character deformations. Landman thinks that the defenses are clothed in pride and created to protect the insecure neurotic from a perceived threatening world. If the patient feels, threatened anger is unleashed. Threats can come, according to Landman, from three directions: from without or interpersonally, from within or intrapsychically, or as a consequence of treatment pressures on the patient to examine, assess and grow.

Landman (1959) sees the idealized image as potentially a vital source of hostility. When its claims are not met, anxiety and the threat of vulnerability occur. The idealized image is nourished by special considerations or entitlements such as deference and attention. If "nourishment" as defined by the patient is not forthcoming, the idealized image unleashes "justified" hostility and/or vindictiveness.

From within or intrapsychically, the character disorder may be frightened of the emergence of the real self in treatment. The conflict between the real self and the pride system then intensifies. Self-doubts, self-hate and hostility also occur to beat back the new, unfamiliar, and therefore threatening, healthy constructive forces.

In terms of interpretative direction, Landman (1959) makes the important point that the patient first needs to connect the hostility with the threatened defensive position. Next, the patient has to feel convinced that he or she can give up the defense, that it is no longer necessary.

THE INTERPRETATION OF SHAME

According to Ward (1972, pp. 62–73), shame can be used defensively to shrug off anxiety-producing material. From a Horneyan perspective there is no doubt that the exposure of what the patient considers shameful would spark intense self-hate. The therapist can employ certain techniques to help the patient expose and therefore be able to work on fantasies that keep him imprisoned in a cramped existence. When the therapist selectively reveals his own unambiguous personal experiences, he is showing the patient that it is possible to feel shame and ultimately live through it.

Also demonstrating that the self-destructive effects of shame are often exaggerated may decrease the shame. It helps if an incident occurs in vivo. Ward (1972) cited such an incident. He had inadvertently scheduled two patients at the same time (I find that this is not an unusual occurrence since almost every therapist sees many patients on a once-per-week basis). One of the patients was an individual who had a lot of trouble dealing with shame. Ward did not try to hide his shame. Ward (p. 71) commented about the incident, "The episode was used in the subsequent hours to illustrate some of the features about witnessing the analyst's shame but [the patient] was impressed and heartened by the fact that it didn't seem as bad as he had anticipated." This incident also gave the patient an opportunity to identify with a man's healthy reference to shame.

Another approach to the patient's fear of exposing shame is to emphasize the price the patient is paying. The therapist's careful revealing of selected aspects of his own personal life relevant to the patient's life may further trust and lessen the anxiety that the patient will be rejected. Ward (1972) especially advocates the helpful procedure of what he terms "explicit labeling of shame ingredients." These are

> the process of hiding parts of the self, the cost of the hiding, the fear of shame, the fears of rejection, the estimates of the chances of rejection on accepting the role of trust, the feeling shame itself, the transitory aspect of the experience of shame, the freedom of energy after revelation and the incorporation of the newly revealed aspect of the self into the rest of the self (p. 73).

The following vignette depicts the interpretation of pride with concomitant shame and the patient's claim to do the impossible.

Barbara began the session by saying that this week was the worst week she had had since she was married. Her stormy marriage was a main issue in therapy so I was expecting that she would detail the latest heated argument between herself and her hot-tempered husband. It seems that she had gone to her best friend's home in a nearby state to pay her respects to her friend who had just lost her grandmother. When she returned home she found her husband was still at work. Feeling tense she decided to drink a little wine. When the husband arrived and kissed her he smelled the alcohol on her breath. He would not accept that she had the wine at home. He vehemently insisted that she had cheated on him. He rushed out into the hallway where he feverishly combed through the garbage to find the wine bottle that the patient claimed was there.

During her husband's tirade, the patient wondered why she even bothered to come home when she was being subjected to so much emotional pain. She asked herself again, "Why am I staying in this terrible marriage?" From the preceding thought she went on to "Why don't I just kill myself? My husband has just told me that I've killed off his ability to love, that I'm a liar, that I disgust him, and that at times he thinks he would like to kill me." She then said to me, "I'll save him the trouble. I'll kill myself." At this point I, feeling some anxiety, reminded her of our contract. She was to call me before she determined to die. The patient had attempted suicide in the past before she came to me and I needed to remind her of our pact. She agreed to stay with her promise.

I recounted at this point the myth of the porcupines. She and her husband were like them in their painful interaction. Like the porcupines who drew closer to each other for warmth, Barbara and her husband stick each other, then draw apart. This dance continues over and over. Barbara voiced how frightened she would feel if she separated and was alone. Besides the patient's problem with attaining healthy autonomy, therapy had revealed that she married to change a type of man who was, like her father, filled with rage. Unlike her father, her husband showed no desire to change. To fail in her mission, her own search for glory, that is, to alter her surrogate husband-father, would be too great a shameful blow to her pride and need to ward off her self-hate.

The next vignette illustrates an interpretative challenge to a patient's self-effacement.

In my office, Irma sparkled with verve, charm, and a delightful, engaging sense of humor. No one, she reported, could put anything over on her, and if they tried they were subjected to her clever, withering, verbal assaults. There was one area though, her work, where she seemed to me and to herself strangely too complacent, too ready to be exploited. She had accepted her present employment with the understanding that she would gain new skills and ultimately earn a respectable salary. Instead her employer repeatedly declined, with lame excuses, to teach her anything new and would not increase her salary despite his loud approval of her talent and work. She, at first, had been eager to gain his approval and respect, but there was no subsequent evident, concrete reward.

Once more Irma was telling me in the session, that in spite of her employer's obvious mistreatment of her, she was going to go along, burying her increasing resentment and discontent. At this point I asked her to tell me what her hopes were when she began working on this job? She readily recounted her heartfelt wish to improve her skills and obtain a decent salary as a result. I then asked, "Would these hopes ever be realized on this job?" "No!," she answered. I sensed that, with my prodding, she was now ready to remember her considerable skills, talents, drive, and desire to learn which her employer was failing to validate and hoping she would forget. She was complying with his "should." Her father had also never recognized her worth and she, caught in self-hate, was not recognizing her own worth as well. Her employer was merely capitalizing on her self-destructive "should," one that said, "Since your father did not recognize your capability, you feel that you should not exercise your rightful claim to recognition of your worth." I was able at this juncture to crystallize her real self's obvious strengths and she could recognize how her employer's "should," pressuring her to be agreeably exploited, was married to her "should," mandating compliant self-effacement.

Irma was galvanized by her new awareness of the destructive consequences of her self-effacement on her job. "I'm going to confront him about his not teaching me and ask for a raise. If I don't get what I deserve,

I will look for another job." The next session she reported that she had confronted her boss in a respectful but determined manner. He held his ground and refused to teach her and grant her a raise. She then informed him that she was quitting, located a headhunter, and was being seriously considered for another higher-paying position.

INTERPRETING TRANSFERENCE, BLOCKAGES, CLAIMS, THE SEARCH FOR GLORY, AND PRIDE

During the course of treatment there are a few sessions which contain almost all the dynamics of a patient's particular "Horneyan" pathology. The following vignette brings out the interpretation of transference, claims, the search for glory, blockages, and pride.

Florence was not happy with the way I had dealt with her report of her family's latest abuse of her in a previous session. What angered her in the session before was that I had told her that she was ignoring the validity of the partial support of her younger sister.

During a very stormy family meeting three of her brothers, the patient and her younger sister were supposed to discuss what could be reasonably done to help their retarded youngest brother significantly improve his living conditions and health.

Florence's oldest brother had in the past physically attacked her during a fierce argument. He had an explosive temper, just like the patient's father, who had physically and sexually abused her as a child. The father, a violent alcoholic, had done the same thing to her other siblings. The patient's mother had masochistically complied with her abusive husband for decades until he assaulted the youngest daughter. She then divorced him.

During the recent family meeting the oldest brother, verbally laced into the patient's sister and her. The two other brothers passively stood by as was their custom and did not intervene. The patient felt a familiar anger toward them for not protecting her from the vitriolic verbal assaults of the brother, emulating her father.

It seemed to me that, like the patient, her younger sister stood up to the raging brother during the meeting and had told him in no uncertain terms that he was chauvinistic, devaluating, and controlling of both her and the patient. I told the patient that she had a prideful claim to be the only one who could stand up to this particularly difficult, infantile brother, just as she was the only one who could confront her father when she was a child. I granted that her sister could have been more explicitly protective of the patient when the brother's anger erupted. Nonetheless the patient was placing an unfair "should" on to her sister as to how she should have better intervened. In addition, the patient was seeking to maintain her idealized image of being the only one who could and would really help her impaired brother. She was seeing her sister transferentially as a function of the past when the patient had truly been the only one in the family to aid her mother during her serious illness. Unlike that time, her sister now, along with the patient, was trying to help ameliorate their brother's plight. I also attempted to help the patient see that her younger sister was hurting and had felt abandoned by the patient, who had gone off to an out-of-town college, leaving the much younger sister unprotected against the tantrums of her sexually abusive father.

Toward the end of the session Florence stated she was no longer angry with me, could experience the truth of what I was suggesting, and could now register more fully her younger sister's partial concern and protection of her. She could also recognize how her rageful brother mirrored her alcoholic father and how her other two brothers' behavior reflected her compliant, passive mother. She determined that she would continue to help her retarded brother but that in the future she would not place herself in a family gathering where she had to face her unstable, abusive older brother=father. In the past, acting out vestiges of self-hate and a need for punishment, the patient had offered herself up to guaranteed pain from her same childish, petulant sibling. During the session I was also able to reach the patient enough so that she could more readily see that she had rejected some of the same interventions I had presented to her during the prior session.

DREAMS

The dream, according to Horney (1958, pp. 222–231), dramatically presents the patient's attempts at a solution to his conflicts. The dream can clarify the patient's ideas and feelings. Dreams can sensitively expose the constructive forces in a patient, promote further understanding, and even offer clues as to whether a patient is ready to end treatment.

Horney (1950a, p. 348) asserts that the main task of the therapist is to utilize the disillusioning process in therapy, thereby reducing the obstructive forces so that the constructive forces of the real self have a chance to flourish. To successfully attain the preceding task (i.e., disillusionment and construction), the therapist needs an extensive understanding of the unconscious complexities within the patient. "To help the patient to find himself the therapist also needs a knowledge to be gained by experience of the ways in which—through dreams and other channels—the real self may emerge" (Horney, p. 348).

Horney (1950a, p. 349) presents the basic tenets of her theory of dreams as follows: "in dreams we are closer to the reality of ourselves; that they represent attempts to solve our conflicts, either in a neurotic or in a healthy way; that in them constructive forces can work, even at a time when they are hardly visible otherwise."

Dreams occasionally can depict a change to a positive attitude. Horney (1950a, p. 359) offers one example of a patient who dreamed of a horse that now limped. But he reasoned in the dream, "I can love him in spite of the limp." This dream heralded a change from self-loathing to feeling "sympathetic toward himself and experiencing himself for the first time as being neither particularly wonderful nor despicable but as the struggling and often harassed human being which he really is" (Horney, p. 359).

Dreams can represent through powerful symbols the character disorder's self-hate and self-contempt when the patient is not conscious of those destructive feelings toward his self (e.g., loathsome insect, dilapidated house).

With regard to various character types, the self-effacing character disorder, for instance, may only become aware that he is tormenting himself or is too readily accepting out of guilt the accusations from others. "His dreams are replete with symbols of self-contempt and self-condemnation" (Horney, 1950a, p. 224). His dreams may also contain executions or he is sentenced to death and he may be uncertain as to why, but he complies. Torture dreams also occur with individuals in the dream who show him no compassion or caring.

The resigned character disorder in their dreams may "reveal a deeply buried sadness, self-hate and hate for others, self-pity, despair, anxiety. In other words there *is* a world of conflicts and passionate feelings under the smooth surface" (Horney, 1950a, p. 289).

The search for glory can be revealed in a dream. Horney (1950a, p. 31) offers an example of a dream of a patient who had a phobia about heights. The dream appeared when he began to question his conviction of indisputable greatness. He dreamed that he was on top of the mountain but he was in peril of falling off. He was holding on desperately to a ridge. Horney (p. 31) understood the dream as meaning that the patient "could not get higher than having (in his mind) a godlike omnipotence and cosmic significance!"

Horney (1942, p. 177) advises that a dream, while it may further understanding, confirm an assumption, provide a needed connection between ideas, or expose a new and surprising direction, may also be hard to read because of blockages.

Adding more valuable clinical observations concerning types of character disorders and their dreams, Horney (1945, p. 80) suggests that the detached character disorder, averse to competition, may reveal in her dreams a hidden treasure which arbiters of taste travel from far and wide to view. The hidden treasure, Horney (p. 80) surmises, is the patient's "intellectual and emotional life which he guards within the magic circle." The opposition of the detached patient to the therapist's effort to help him change the status quo will be revealed in dreams in the following manner: "the analytical situation may appear as a long distance call between two reporters on different continents" (Horney, p. 87). Horney concludes that this dream represents the patient's desire to keep the entire treatment process removed from her.

Horney (1945, p. 80) comments on the role of externalization in dreams. She offers an example of a dream of a patient where the therapist is pictured as a "jailer," but the actual "jailer" was the patient himself.

Therapists, according to Horney (1956b, p. 203), need to pay particular attention to the feeling aspect in a dream. She points out that a dream may expose a surprising passion in a seemingly unfeeling individual. Horney (p. 203) advises that "We must rely on the understanding of the patient which we obtain by feeling ourselves into his situation to determine whether or not we should communicate what his dreams reveal." She cautions the therapist to desist from communicating the meaning of a dream when the therapist has a feeling within himself that warns the therapist that the patient is not ready to confront the meaning of his dreams. In this case the therapist "must be guided by our intuitive understanding of the patient's capacity to take in that which may still be too upsetting to his shaky equilibrium" (Horney, p. 203).

Horney distinguishes her basic view of dreams from that of Freud. She writes "Whereas Freud called the dream the royal road to the unconscious, I see it as the royal way to the truth of ourselves." She felt that dreams represent a mending process—which disables neurotic positions and furthers the silent emergence of self-realizing tendencies.

> We can interpret many dreams as though the real self of the dreamer were saying to him "Look how you despise yourself! Look what you are doing to yourself, how you are divided, what phantoms you are chasing, what a crooked path you are following, what a foul compromise you are trying to make!" (Horney, 1958, p. 227).

In the case of self-hating dreams in which the idealized self may be perceiving the real self with disdain, Horney (p. 227) advises that the best interpretation is one in which the therapist includes both the constructive and destructive aspects of the character structure. Inclusion of the disquieting pressure (e.g., anxiety, conflict, urge to be more liberated from neurotic constraints) responsible for the dream needs to be understood and interpreted.

Horney (1958, pp. 229–231) offers specific approaches to the analysis of the dream. Beginning with an overall view, she suggests that the therapist strive for a general understanding of the dream, followed by attention to the details, the stimulus (the disquieting elements) for the dream, and the nature of the accompanying solution.

Whatever the patient said in the session may be connected to the dream. The therapist considers the character trends and conflicts in the dream and relates them to the patient's life. There is no need to keep trying to understand a dream if all attempts fail. Later sessions may shed light on the dream. When there is an absence of associations to a patient's dream a specific question is the best approach, such as "Is there any part of the dream which made you think of something?" or "Choose a specific symbol or theme and connect it with those of previous dreams" (Horney, 1958, p. 230).

Horney (1958, p. 230) suggests other questions about the dream: "Feelings in the dream; 'Are the feelings in the dream appropriate to the dream?' 'How is the dreamer symbolized? What is his goal? How far is he removed from himself'" (Horney, 1958, p. 230); the passivity or activity of the dreamer; the action in the dream; the role of the dreamer. "What is the attitude of the dreamer toward other figures in the dream? Is he distant, close, compliant, suspicious? Does he show much feeling for himself, or is he a spectator of the dream, regarding it as though it were a piece of fiction" (Horney, 1958, p. 230).

Horney (1958, p. 230) presents a dream of a patient and its handling by an analyst that best illustrate an important consideration in fully understanding the dream and the dreamer. The patient, who had gotten more in touch with her pride, dreamed that she was traveling with her mother, a woman enamored with prestige. They were going to visit an individual whose predominate character trait was open-heartedness. Horney reports that the analyst, by allowing himself to feel into the dream, accurately interpreted the patient's visit to the warm individual as a moving away from her mother's shallow values, once thought of by the patient as strength by contrast to values that really matter.

Finally, Horney (1958, p. 231) reminds the therapist never to forget consideration of the constructive aspects of the dream; what is really constructive and just how beneficial. Horney (p. 231) further refines in a valuable manner how constructiveness in the dream needs to be scrutinized by the therapist. As she (Horney, p. 231) writes,

> Awareness of neurotic qualities is not constructive if the patient still invests pride in them. A patient may acknowledge his deceitfulness but still defend or glorify it. Awareness of neurotic qualities becomes constructive when the patient experiences disgust in the dream, and asks, in a sudden awakening, "What am I doing to myself?" Dreams are also constructive when a patient takes a stand or deals with anxiety or conflict.

THE WORKING ALLIANCE

Horney's vision of the "working alliance" or the nature of the therapist's helping role is that he establishes a setting of friendly interest. What is important is that "the simple fact that the analyst wants to understand the patient implies that he takes him seriously" (Horney, 1942, p. 144). The therapist "through his own attitude inspires the courage to be on friendly terms with oneself" (Horney, p. 144). When the therapist attempts to engage in understanding and a battle to reduce the patient's conflicts and anxieties, the patient feels encouraged and emotionally supported. Most importantly, having the therapist the patient feels better because "he needs someone who does not lose faith in him, even though his own faith is gone (Horney, p. 145).

Horney (1946a, pp. 106–109) delineates the basic elements of the helping relationship established by the therapist. She underscores the therapist's willingness to understand and

> his unflagging interest in the patient's growth, his faith in the patient's existing potentialities, his firmness that permits him to view the patient's sufferings with concern without letting himself be crushed by them, to remain unswayed by the patient's admiration and undaunted by the patient's aggressive demands or hostile attacks (Horney, 1946a, p. 106).

Another good supporting factor enforcing the working alliance is "the analyst's consistent emphasis on what he believes to be the patient's best interests" (Horney, 1946a, p. 107). This does not mean that the therapist is despotic or authoritative but that he "endeavors to find out together with the patient in what manner he is blocking his own way" (Horney, 1946a, p. 107). The therapist, according to Horney (pp. 108–109), recognizes that it is vital for an individual to assume responsibility for himself. The therapist knows that each individual is unique and needs to make decisions in terms of his own wishes, needs, and values. The therapist remembers that behavior is too complex for him to give advice and so he has realistic humility; he is aware of his limitations. The humble attitude of the therapist does not preclude the possibility that "he may definitely advise against a major decision if he is convinced that the patient is acting under the pressure of irrational emotional forces" (Horney, p. 108).

Finally, Horney (1946, p. 108) presents a startling observation which is that, contrary to what most people might assume, "the patient is not interested in himself as he *is*. He is constantly concerned with what he *should* be and blames himself for his shortcomings instead of tackling them realistically." The therapist, believing in the constructive forces within the patient, consistently interested in the patient, being tolerant, interpreting, explaining, and questioning, advances the helping, cooperative process; consequently the patient obtains insight into his mind and ends up in the "driver's seat" with regard to his life.

A proper therapeutic attitude, one that will endorse a good working alliance, is presented by Martin (1966). He urges therapists to keep their eye constantly on the constructive forces within the patient. We are cautioned not to tell a patient how to lead his life but to help the patient become more cognizant as to the nature of the life he is leading. The patient discloses areas to be worked on, what his priority is. We can tell the patient where to explore but we can not tell the patient what he will find or hear. Using the patient's own language, his terms, we show respect for the patient's inner world. We help the patient develop constructive listening to himself. Martin (p. 285) suggests that "Emphasis on the healthy aspect of the patient is implied when you keep broadening the context, when you elicit more and more of the 'what' that is happening and 'what else is going on' before you ask 'why.'"

If the patient says "I am depressed," for example, it is better to inquire as to how it shows itself, or to ask "What is being depressed," or "What else is happening?"

I foster the working alliance by letting the patient know why I ask certain questions. At times when it is relevant, I tell the patient that sometimes it is difficult to talk about certain matters but it is helpful if she tries to be as open a possible. I reassure the patient that I will readily admit an error but will ask the patient how they feel about my mistake and my admission. I suggest to the patient that he ask periodically how our work is progressing or stumbling. I state that I, in turn, will tell him how I feel about his assessment of our progress.

I inform the patient that when I do not fully understand the significant meaning of his utterance in a session, I will always seek to understand what he is trying to really communicate. I emphasize that together we will find out what it was about. I offer the patient my admiration for working on a difficult and painful task of exposing herself to me.

I convey to the patient by my attitude and words that I accept the patient's ability to develop insight at her own pace. I emphasize to the patient that, as they speak, they should try to scan the meaning of their verbalizations. This will help them to grasp how what they are saying will help them to understand themselves and their problems better.

Above all else I keep in mind the ultimate goal of therapy annunciated by Horney (1950a, p. 157).

> It is the aim of character analysis to help people achieve a greater inner freedom so that they may grow as human beings. Self-realization is of great importance—realization on the part of the patient of what he really feels and wants, rather than what he thinks he should feel and want; realization also of the ability to tap his own resources, gradually to assume responsibility for himself, to develop constructive relationships with others, to do productive and meaningful work, to develop whatever special gifts he may have.

9   Transference and Counter-Transference

TRANSFERENCE

When Horney (1917) wrote about the topic of transference, she was still adhering mainly to classical Freudian psychoanalysis. In her paper "The Technique of Psychoanalytic Therapy" (1917), she states that transference is mostly positive but, after a length of time, it may become a vehicle of powerful resistance (e.g., embarrassment causing reluctance to voice thoughts, feelings, or fantasies thought bad).

Although written in 1935, during the early formative development of psychoanalytic concepts, Horney's paper "On the Difficulties in Dealing with the Transference" (1935b) defines transference and clearly traces its main implications for treatment.

Horney introduces her ideas in the paper by first noting that the therapist deals with potentially explosive issues when treating patients. It is bewildering when, in spite of the best efforts of the therapist, the patient reacts with opposition, rejection, irritation, contempt, and sarcasm. Complicating the expression of all these preceding negative responses, the patient may have no conscious awareness that he is behaving in an obstructive fashion. Sometimes the obstruction may take the form of the patient becoming excessively dependent on the therapist, and no amount of effort on the therapist's part appears to reduce the dependency. When these obstructive forces in the session occur, the therapist, according to

Horney, may be thrown off balance and become uncertain as to how to deal effectively with the patient's negative, disruptive response. Horney (1935b, p. 53) credits Freud with the discovery that these negative reactions are not only stimulated by present events in the treatment but by early childhood experiences. Horney (p. 53) cites Freud's view where "He called these reactions 'transference' because the patient often seemed to revive certain attitudes toward persons of the early environment and to 'transfer' them to the analyst."

Horney puts forth the idea that transference reactions occur outside the treatment room. All it takes to trigger a transference response is anxiety. Transference, whether it is positive, such as admiration toward the therapist, or negative, such as scorn or sarcasm, is always unrealistic and irrational.

Occasionally, the fact that the therapist points out to the patient that his behavior reflected a significant childhood relationship, such as, "You are angry with me just as you were toward your brother," may mildly benefit the patient. However, Horney points out that this transference interpretation to the patient has limited value since it is largely intellectually based.

We can see in Horney's early paper (1935b) her beginning emphasis on the significance of the present in dealing with transference and other issues. She raises for consideration what makes a patient who has been spoiled, for instance, continue to express transferentially an excessive demand for immoderate attention from the therapist. Horney (p. 55) states

> Self-evident as it is, it seems necessary in the face of certain misunderstandings to emphasize that the therapeutic aim in psychoanalytic therapy or any kind of treatment akin to it is *not* to recapture childhood memories, but to change something in the present attitudes.

The patient's transference responses offer the therapist the best glimpse and conviction of the patient's character trends. Horney (p. 55) offers an example of a patient who becomes easily infuriated when someone has let her down or failed to fulfill a duty toward her. The therapist can have the hypothesis that the patient may be making inordinate demands and, when the individual does not meet her perfectionistic standards, the patient becomes righteously indignant and enraged because of her disappointment.

But the therapist's hypothesis is best verified when the patient overreacts with rage because she had to wait 10 minutes beyond her usual session appointment.

Horney (1935b, p. 56) cautions that the therapist should not allow transference emotions to accumulate without the therapist exposing them to the patient when they come up. She (Horney, p. 56) warns that if they are neglected, "the patient's affect will accumulate and not only cause him suffering which might have been avoided, but also render it extremely difficult to cope with." Horney (p. 56) mentions a number of common examples of transference reactions: the patient who is angry because the session is limited in frequency and time, because the therapist is not omniscient, because the patient finds the therapist is a mere mortal and not perfect, or because the therapist does not give the patient as much affection as the patient believes he requires. Horney (pp. 52–58) counsels that the therapist needs to be active in exposing transference manifestations, because the patient will usually not spontaneously volunteer that he is expressing a transference wish and/or affect. Toward the end of her paper, Horney (pp. 57–58) presents the kernel of her thinking on the best way to handle a patient's transference. She states

> As a rule a patient will willingly admit that he is spiteful toward the analyst as he was toward his father, but it will require all the analyst's observation, energy and consistency to prove to the patient that he is spiteful just now because he has not complied with his demand to see him three times a week instead of twice or with whatever demands he may have had.

Horney continued to develop her thinking regarding transference and her 1935 papers reflect the embryonic beginnings of her final theory and technique.

In Horney's paper (1935a) "Concepts and Misconcepts of the Analytic Method," she shows an inclination to draw away from the classical treatment of the transference when she downgrades the importance of the historical genesis of the transference. She adopts, based on her increased clinical experience, a pragmatic point of view. She declares that what counts is a full description of what the transference is and how it enfolds toward the therapist. Going more completely into the negative consequences of the transference, Horney moves therapy forward in a fruitful direction. Immediate factors determining present attitudes have to be noted and interpreted (e.g., the dutiful patient who transfers his submissiveness, and the need for the therapist to bring this characterological trait to the patient's awareness).

Horney (1935a) leaves out the transference of historical antecedents and stresses the value of interpreting the patient's surface attitudes. She presents an instance of a patient idealizing the therapist, shown by a wish to please and appease, the bringing in of lengthy dreams and fascinating childhood material. Although Horney does not explicitly say so, she implies that the classical Freudian approach linking idealization to the transference of idealized parental figures would not be as productive as the interpretation of the surface attitudes of detachment and aloofness. I would supplement her well-founded advice by adding counter-transference to the transference mix. A narcissistic therapist who unconsciously desires to be idealized would want and encourage a worshipful attitude. Similarly the aloof therapist uncomfortable with powerful affects would unconsciously promote detachment.

In Horney's paper (1935b) "On Difficulties in Dealing with the Transference," she explicitly allows her discontent with the classical approach to transference to emerge. It is the scrutiny of the "what" and "how" and the "here and now" of the patient's transference that really counts as the chief ameliorative therapeutic element. I think that Horney's more comfortable and pronounced shift away from the classical treatment model had a lot to do with Melanie Klein's influence, for Horney uses as evidence of her new way of thinking, the manifestation of the patient's envy. The understanding of envy was and is a basic component of Kleinian therapy. The "here and now" treatment of envy is central to Kleinian analysis but, unlike Horney, Kleinians postulate very primitive, infantile transferential elements.

Horney (1935b) at this stage of her theory development does caution the therapist to deal early with transference and not to let it accumulate, so as to siphon off bottled-up resentments and disruptive anxiety.

A good or "on target" interpretation of transference attitudes or other aspects of a patient's character structure may elicit a desire to compete with the therapist, as if the therapist has scored some points by perceiving something the patient has not seen. There may be disparagement and, beneath awareness, a disguised anger. Horney (1935b) points out that there is a type of individual in our society who can be intensely competitive and have a huge ego. She goes on to describe what she has called the expansive character disorder (i.e., expecting perfection, wishing to be unique, implicitly envious or fearful of being envied and hypersensitive to criticism or what are seen as accusations, and desiring idealized admiration).

The following vignette is that of Edward, a patient who illustrates a powerful, dramatic, disruptive transference blockage precipitating a very quick termination of treatment by the patient. What the patient said in his first and what was to be his last session is noteworthy because it shows so well the pretense of admiration toward the therapist. It is somewhat akin to enacting the modified advice of an experienced comic, that is, "Always leave them laughing." Although in this case it was "Always leave them (i.e., the therapist) feeling as if they were an admired and exceptional person."

The patient, Edward, said at the end of the first session, "You are the most intelligent man I ever met," and that was the last time I saw him. He baffled and frustrated me. Since it was at the end of the session as he was closing my office door, I did not have a chance to explore with him just what he meant or intended by his gushing compliment. My hunch was that he fled treatment because he was concerned about becoming anxious. If he'd stayed he would inevitably have had to confront his possible manipulative maneuvers, an alienation of many intimates, and the chief basis for his entering treatment in the first place.

The best reaction to a transference interpretation, or again any interpretation, is relief and a more successful adaptation and resolution of problems.

Horney (1935b) ends her paper by emphasizing in no uncertain terms that the therapist should deal with what she sees as the "upper," surface levels of the patient's behavior, or what I term the "significant obvious," to obtain the greatest progress in therapy.

COUNTER-TRANSFERENCE

Horney (1957a) develops her understanding of the vital element of counter-transference in her paper "The Analyst's Personal Equation." Counter-transference is the blocking of the therapist's competence by his own character disorder deformations. The therapist, Horney (1935b) strongly advises, needs to perpetually monitor his work and strive to increase his competence. Monitoring his competence is difficult because there is a need on the part of the therapist to see his therapeutic capability as quite satisfactory. Certain types of patients (e.g., the self-effacing character disorder) flatter the therapist's idealized image by overestimating his significance in their life. Horney (1935b) points out that the expansive, aggressive patient may get under the aggressive therapist's skin by hurting his vulnerable spot—pride. The narcissistic therapist will also be emotionally vulnerable as a consequence of overvaluing himself. Every neurotic, sensitive part of the therapist is a potential source of counter-transference. The therapist, for example, who is anxious about his neurotic conflict emerging will treat the patient's issues in a gingerly fashion.

Horney (1957a, pp. 194–197) divides the therapist along six character disorder lines and describes the usual or frequent counter-transferences associated with each of them.

The compliant therapist has a compulsive directive to be liked. He stresses the patient's assets and minimizes any displays of hostility. He is fearful of angering the patient and avoids interpreting the patient's idealized image. He may be too giving regarding his fees and times. He is too sympathetic and concerned with making the patient too dependent on him. The therapist will tend to overemphasize empathy and identification, seeing therapy too much from the patient's viewpoint.

The aggressive therapist can be controlling, insensitive, and injure the patient's feelings. He may "shoot from the hip," interpret dynamics too quickly, be dogmatic and omniscient.

The narcissistic therapist generalizes too much, types his patients, and does not free himself from stereotyped perceptions. He feels either impotent and/or hopeless if the patient rejects his interpretation. He has convinced himself that he is the only one who can help the patient change.

The perfectionistic therapist is tenacious and detail-oriented but overlooks the big picture, the main priority. He is didactic, controlling, and relatively insensitive to the patient's feelings. He is dominated by "shoulds" and at times may berate himself for not being the "perfect" therapist.

The arrogant-vindictive therapist is not sufficiently compassionate. He is self-serving and self-righteous. He tends to foster dependency.

The detached or resigned therapist predominantly observes and does not experience sufficient feelings. He is made anxious by a potential involvement so he avoids evoking strong feelings. He can easily slip into hopelessness as he believes change seldom takes place. He is impatient and wants quick results (e.g., supervisee who desired an instant, magical cure of a patient's worry over a dreaded malpractice suit, and at the same time asserted that patients really do not change).

To facilitate awareness of counter-transference, Horney (1957a), as it has been mentioned before, strongly suggests that the therapist always try to arrive at the feeling by closely connecting with the point in the session that triggers off a counter-transference. The therapist needs to ask himself, "Is this an appropriate feeling I am having in reaction to what the patient is saying and/or doing?"

In conclusion, Horney (1957a, p. 197) advises therapists, "A constant effort to examine our reactions and even our associations and to relate them to what is going on in the patient is essential if we are to help the patient toward self-realization and to keep growing ourselves."

10 Verbatim Treatment Selections

In this chapter I will illustrate the utilization of the basic processes of Horneyan psychotherapy: disillusionment and construction. I shall cover four sessions that touch on all of the major problems that beset a specific patient, Martha.

The patient entered therapy because she was anxious and depressed about her health, distrust of men, poor relationship with her daughter, worry about her daughter's marriage, envy of her sister, and difficulty dealing with her alcoholic ex-husband.

Fortunately the patient spoke slowly so that I was able to record easily and attend without distraction to our verbal interchange. I did not have to depend on my memory, which might have caused me to omit significant therapy issues. Verbatim note-taking can capture the essence and nuances of the dynamics of each session. The verbatim selections are equivalent to inviting the reader as a spectator into the treatment room.

During the four sessions, I worked with the patient to weaken the obstructive forces within her character structure and gave her blocked real self the opportunity to flourish. I shall also comment about the dynamics underlying each of the patient's statements and the rationale of my interventions.

SESSION TWO

MARTHA: *I'm afraid to baby sit my new grandchild. I worry about having a heart attack.*

A good example of Horney's idea of basic anxiety in this case because the anxiety acts as a lever to expose a sector of the patient's pathology that needs attention. Martha is concerned that something bad will happen within her that will harm the baby. Martha represents the threatening, unsafe environment. Perhaps her statement expresses a possible eruption of sadistic impulses but evidence is required to substantiate the validity of this hypothesis.

ME: *What makes you think that that will happen?*

Although I think I know her reasons for concern (i.e., a previous heart attack), I always believe that it is best for the patient to express their own fantasies in back of any comment they make. Sometimes very valuable, surprising material emerges.

MARTHA: *I have been experiencing pains.*

ME: *You've had recent medical examinations that showed that you did not have any problem with your heart. You told me in the first session that your heart surgery had been very successful.*

MARTHA: *True. I suppose my medical training as a nurse increases my imagination, which is running wild.*

Her basic anxiety causes her to see her body on the verge of betraying her. Given her medical training, she can readily supply the details of an impending, disastrous heart attack. Since I suffered a near-fatal heart attack and bypass surgery, I can readily empathize with a certain reality of her concern.

ME: *Is there anything else keeping your anxiety going?*

I sensed that her past heart attack and her medical training, while part of her basic anxiety, were not the entire story. There seemed to be an underlying mistrust of the consistent medical reassurances given to her by her doctors, who emphatically told her she was now okay. I know that if self-hate is present it will continue to make its appearance by not allowing any good to come in the form of reassurance. She will continue to see herself as damaged.

MARTHA: *I don't trust men. I've had bad experiences with them. My ex-husband, boyfriends, and the many arrogant doctors I have worked with.*

Her bad past experiences have left her with the claim that she is entitled to distrust all men. In addition, her distrust causes her to feel anxiety about her body and sustain suffering. Her sadistic impulses appear to have turned against her body. I decide to deal first with her claim. I file away the thought that I'm eventually going to have to deal with her feelings about me as another man she might not be able to trust, that is, a negative transference issue.

ME: *Are you saying all men can't be trusted?*

MARTHA: *Not all, just most.*

A qualified retreat but the claim of distrust is still held. I am heartened by the qualification, which means that her real self recognizes that there are men, possibly including me, who can be trusted. The transference of distrust, I gauge, is not strong enough to be dealt with now.

I turn to another more immediate problem. I remember that Martha is using her nursing skills taking care of a very ill, aged mother of a friend. She does not seem anxious about having a fatal heart attack while nursing this very ill woman.

Perhaps I can use this knowledge to weaken her anxiety about her body and brooding torment.

ME: *You don't seem worried about having a fatal heart attack taking care of a very sick woman of advanced age.*

What is she going to say about this contradiction?

MARTHA: *I know it may not seem to make sense but I get a lot out of taking care of her.*

What she gets is still unknown but it is obviously enough to markedly reduce her worry and anxiety about her heart condition.

ME: *So what does it do for you taking care of her?*

I'm attempting to zero in on what she feels that allows her to successfully deal with a stressful situation, a very sick, very elderly adult. This confidence does not seem to carry over to her daughter's newborn child.

MARTHA: *The 90-year-old mother treats me with more respect than she treats her own daughter.*

Competition enters here, with Martha as the "daughter" triumphing over another daughter. In Martha's case the elderly woman's daughter is transferentially seen by her as an older sister. Martha is transferentially contending with her sister for mother's approval. I decide to interpret the competition but not the transference, as this is only the second session, too early in treatment, and competition is closer to the surface.

ME: *You beat out the daughter and that seems to make you feel good.*

I introduce the competitive factor and choose to leave out the pride factor for another, later examination.

MARTHA: *I see what you mean about the competition.*

Martha is becoming more aware and accepting of the possibility that she is competing with her patient's daughter. I see that she may be more willing to pursue further details of the competitive nature of her character structure.

ME: *Do you suppose that you are worried that you will not receive the same kind of approval from your daughter when you watch your new grandchild?*

I throw out the possibility that Martha's daughter, unlike the elderly patient, will not value Martha comparably and will repeat what Martha experienced as a child when her mother clearly favored her older sister. (I surmised this occurrence in the first session.)

MARTHA: *It's hard to please my daughter. She is so demanding and critical.*

While it is possible that her daughter is demanding and critical there is also the possibility that the patient is "externalizing," to use Horney's term, and is projecting her own characterological features on to her daughter, that is, her own demandingness and criticality.

ME: *What made you volunteer to babysit so extensively for your daughter in the first place?*

I asked this question to understand with Martha what motivated her to make such a generous offer, given her anxiety about her heart. Perhaps there is another part of her true self emerging here, a constructive force. This is an example of how a therapist utilizes the Horneyan model to disillusion, such as helping the patient become aware of her competitiveness, and at the same time trying to bring to the surface a latent, constructive ingredient of her true self.

MARTHA: *I thought about the joy I would feel when I held my first grandchild.*

The patient's real self and her constructive potency makes its appearance. She declares her capacity to feel genuine jubilation when she gives love to another human being.

SESSION THREE

MARTHA: *My ex-husband showed up at my house. He was drunk as usual.*

I recall that she had informed me in the first session that her ex-husband was an alcoholic and would appear suddenly every now and then without any prior warning. Despite the divorce he would not let go of his conviction that he was still married to Martha.

ME: *So what happened?*

MARTHA: *I called his girlfriend and she came for him. I think he thinks that I can take better care of him than her.*

Maybe it's true. But there is also competition with the girlfriend appearing again, with Martha the "winner." I decide to bring rivalry to her attention.

ME: *You sound like you are competing with her.*

MARTHA: *No competition! I win "hands down." She is a selfish bitch and doesn't really care about anybody.*

This is where you, the reader, had to be there but I sensed a pride in her strong declaration.

ME: *You seem to be proud of just how much you care.*

I'm attempting to help her get in touch with her idealized image, which appears to be striving to be the ultimate successful rescuer.

MARTHA: *I care too much about the wrong men and I seem to pick losers. All my boyfriends, including my ex-husband, were alcoholics.*

Her idealized image as a rescuer maintains self-hate by picking damaged men whom she inevitably can not save.

ME: *But you have been and are a good mother to your daughter and your son.*

I know my declaration to be true from my impression of the quality of her mothering gained during the first session. I want to leave her with deserved good feelings about her self to offset the destructive self-hate possibly released by her failed attempts to save the self-destructive men in her life.

MARTHA: *I've worked at it under the most trying conditions. An alcoholic husband, financial stresses, and being a full-time mother and father. Working too. And I want to be there for my daughter and my new grandchild.*

The patient becomes a compassionate and correct historian of her great accomplishments. Self-hate is aborted.

SESSION FOUR

MARTHA: *I've been concerned about my daughter's choice of husband.*

I wonder if the patient is now directing her disappointment with men toward her son-in-law.

ME: *How's that?*

MARTHA: *He's passive and lacks ambition. My daughter is very ambitious and successful in her career.*

Is she using her daughter as a way of competing with her daughter's husband? I decide to test out this hypothesis.

ME: *It seems to me that, in contrasting your daughter with her husband to his detriment, you are in a sense competing with him as a man by saying that your daughter who represents you is superior to him.*

MARTHA: *I don't know about the competitive part but I have been bad-mouthing him to my daughter.*

Martha is creating potential trouble in her daughter's marriage, a possible future source of suffering and guilt for herself. If her daughter is fired up by the patient she may act out her mother's rivalry with men by creating marital strife. Martha out of guilt alone will experience intensified self-hate and depression.

ME: *How does your daughter see her husband?*

I want to put on the table another "reality" perspective: what does her daughter think about her husband? This is to highlight and contrast if possible the patient's "should" regarding hostility toward men that would urge her to damage her daughter's marriage.

Of course, if her daughter feels the same way as Martha does toward her husband, it would be very difficult to deal with the patient's "should" as distorted, thus transferentially distorting reality.

MARTHA: *She thinks that he could be more ambitious but on the whole she loves him.*

The good outweighs the bad. Her daughter has a more nuanced view of her husband than Martha does.

ME: *Do you suppose you might allow your daughter to come to her own independent judgment about her husband?*

I offer her another "should," one that is, I think, healthier than Martha's need to compete with men. The healthy "should" I present is one which says "It's best not to allow your distorted attitudes to poison the most significant relation of your daughter."

This "should" is essentially more appropriately respectful of her daughter's autonomy as an adult.

MARTHA: *I have already begun to back off from sharing any bad thoughts I have about my son-in-law.*

ME: *What made you change your mind?*

I want to know what made her change her tactics. I also can check the strength of our alliance and quite possibly reinforce a healthy "should," namely, allowing her daughter to form her own conclusions about her husband.

MARTHA: *I want to be a better mother to my daughter than my mother was to me.*

I remain silent as the patient was spontaneously introducing a vital part of her history that she had touched on in the initial session. I noted, of course, her constructive desire to let her real self emerge by contrast to her mother's controlling, interfering, pathological character structure.

MARTHA: *My mother ignored me and just wanted to please my sister.*

ME: *I sense some anger at your mother and perhaps some envy toward your sister for her favored status with your mother.*

I clearly saw her anger at her mother but I hedged my intervention with "perhaps" about anger toward her sister. Let's see what she does with her feelings toward her sister.

MARTHA: *I took after my father while my sister was more like my mother.*

ME: *That might explain why your mother wanted to please your sister more than she wished to please you and that must have hurt.*

An easy interpretation based on the idea that we tend to feel closer toward those individuals more like ourselves. I left the envy of her sister alone for the moment. I wanted Martha to know that I recognized her hurt.

MARTHA: *I did feel sad then but I also remember that my sister was like a "little mother" to me.*

Alongside her anger and envy toward her sister, Martha also felt loving toward her. Apparently the sister was a surrogate, nourishing mother to her. The patient could now get in touch with an appropriate gratitude related to her sister, a gratitude originating from her healthy, constructive real self.

SESSION FIVE

MARTHA: *The last session about my sister brought back a lot of feelings I used to have and maybe still have toward her.*

ME: *What sort of feelings?*

I wanted her to elaborate on her feelings but I also noticed the blockage in the use of the word "maybe."

MARTHA: *I envy her wealth and, unlike me, she still has a husband.*

ME: *Is she really that much better off than you?*

I asked this question with a skeptical tone. My experience with other patients has demonstrated with regard to envy that invariably the one envied is endowed with the patient's externalization of glory that is not at all in keeping with reality.

MARTHA: *Well, her husband is an alcoholic and her kids have not turned out so well.*

My skeptical question has produced some good results, the puncturing of the basis of Martha's envy, the unreal endowment of glory to the envied one.

Still my ex-husband is still in the picture. He showed up with the pretext of wanting to speak to me about my daughter. He frightened me, telling me that our son had had an accident. It was so distorted because it was an accident our son had had 6 years ago. He made it sound like another accident had happened now. He was saying it this way so he could frighten me, into wanting to see and talk to him.

ME: *If he upsets you so much so frequently why do you continue to see him?*

I explore with her why her self-hate requires her to invite guaranteed pain. Is she so alienated from her self-hate that she relinquishes appropriate self-protection from her destructive ex-husband? I decide I would offer her an interpretation dealing with her lack of trust in her real self's good capacity to steer clear of assured, potential suffering.

MARTHA: *He did sound drunk on the phone.*

ME: *Is it possible that you claim to have exceptional ability to deal productively when challenged by a man who is quite drunk?*

I extend my previous intervention by bringing up a possible claim in the service of her idealized image and her search for glory, that is, claiming unique, communicative power and rescuing talents.

MARTHA: *No, I realize now that I should have hung up on him when I heard him slurring his words.*

At last a healthy "should" and the end of the session but not the end of therapy, which continued for 2 more years on a once-per-week basis.

When Martha ended treatment she was a vital part of her grandchild's life, had a significantly better relationship with her daughter, son-in-law, and sister. Her husband had died and Martha had been his nurse the last week of his life. She had not seen or talked to him until the time he entered the hospital. As she put it, "I put away the last drop of possible guilt regarding him by being there for him at the end."

11 Summary of Main Elements and Ending Therapy

SUMMARY OF THE MAIN ELEMENTS OF HORNEYAN PSYCHOTHERAPY

Karen Horney (1945, 1950a) presented her overview of the essential elements of Horneyan therapy in two chapters, each one at the end of her two major works, *Our Inner Conflicts* (1945) and *Neurosis and Human Growth* (1950a). In *Our Inner Conflicts* Horney addresses the challenging task of altering a patient's conflicts. She quickly disposes of the idea that mere insight or knowledge of the genesis of the pathology is sufficient to change character pathology. She finds that formidable blockages occur, such as intellectualization, denial, minimization, despair, fantasies of omnipotence, or transferential blockages, such as, "the therapist is perceived as incompetent."

In *Neurosis and Human Growth* (1950a), the therapist, according to Horney, should be guided by a number of goals. These are the reduction of alienation, increasing the patient's freedom of choice and values, and greater capacity to adapt using his feelings and convictions. The therapist attends to all the patient's solutions and their results. He examines the particular idealized image and specific externalizations. He aids the patient in spotting how the solutions play out in terms of attitudes, constraints, and compromises in the patient's life. He expects to find, throughout the process of exploration, blockages and transferences which are repeatedly interpreted.

159

Before the therapist interprets he employs two criteria: the intervention probably can be taken in by the patient and it is not injurious.

The therapist will not be successful if he tackles significant conflicts without exposing the deleterious consequences in the patient's life. The idealized image, very real in its capacity to fend off self-hate and possibly the "glue" that holds the patient together, should be approached cautiously. The same caution holds true for sadistic trends. They are usually considered too "evil" to be acknowledge or owned by patient.

The aggressive character structure will most likely not appreciate any interpretation that exposes a hint of weakness, a need for intimacy, or possible hopelessness. Despair would represent a defeatist self-pity.

The compliant character disorder does not welcome any recognition of vindictiveness or desire for power.

A rigid idealized self-image coupled with externalization resists interpretations, but knowledge of the patient's pseudo-solutions can give the therapist clues to various not-so-obvious aspects of the patient's character disorder. Therapeutic intuition and sensitivity is, of course, indispensable. How the patient reacts to an interpretation tells us when the patient is repeatedly able to work on and through a problem.

Working through consists of a steady sequence of objectives. First, there is the bringing to the patient's awareness all the obvious and less observable facets of a trend, idealized image, and so forth. Second, inviting the patient to let in its compulsive makeup, and third, promoting an appreciation of the trend's solutions and so forth, their importance to the patient, and their negative results.

Horney enjoins the therapist to concentrate on the nature of the character structure deformation and the blockage preserving it before looking at how it is manifested. The patient needs to realize how much a specific character limitation operates in his life. Usually the negative character attitude serves to ward off or balance another pathological predisposition, such as fantasies of omnipotence subduing excessive fears of failure. Much is gained when the patient is helped to see the opposite side of the coin; it strengthens the working alliance. Helping the patient get in touch with all the ways he perceives the status quo, such as lacerating self-criticism, enhances his healthy determination to change.

In the event that therapy stalls, the therapist must look at the degree of hopelessness, competitive need to defeat the therapist, blaming outside factors, need to experience continued omnipotence, fear of supposed "weakness."

Horney (1945) suggests that hidden hostility usually surfaces as irritability. Diminished helplessness to deal with perceived threats reduces hostility and increases the patient's increased self-esteem. Improvement is shown by the patient's greater friendliness and involvement with others and himself. The patient will obtain a greater capacity to take responsibility for himself and others. Inner independence, a valuable establishment of one's own ladder of values, and respect for the individuality of others make their desirable appearance. The patient sincerely feels more alive, spontaneous, with a sharpened capacity to love without morbid dependency or sadistic control. Horney concludes with one very important caveat to the therapist, which is that he not be captured too strongly by any of the enumerated desirable goals. No patient can become a perfect being.

TERMINATION

Termination, the ending of therapy, is inescapably intertwined with the aims of therapy. Broadly speaking, in "Self-Analysis" (1942) Horney laid down three basic goals: (1) recognize character trends, (2) explore their implications, and (3) see all the relationships between the trends.

Horney (1946b) corrects a common misunderstanding regarding patients who have completed therapy. She (Horney, p. 110) makes the point that the patient's

> growth as a human being, however, is a process that can and should go on as long as you live. Hence analysis as a means of gaining self-knowledge is intrinsically an interminable process. Analytical therapy, while it helps you to disentangle yourself from the web of conflicts and to develop a sounder basis only initiates this development, it does not and cannot complete it.

Successful completion of therapy initiates and institutes a methodology within the patient that allows him to deal more competently with future conflicts and emotional stresses. I have seen the workings of this internalized therapeutic introspection when I have had patients return on occasion for brief periods of time. The patient may say "I heard your voice in my head and questions you would have asked and that helped me deal better with the problem."

Since we are dealing with the whole personality structure, that is, the character disorder, according to Horney (1946b) it is much more difficult to decide when the patient is ready to leave treatment. Horney offers some basic criteria for termination. The patient should become more flexible, less easily hurt, less self-important, more confident, and have his feet firmly on the ground. More precisely, "when can the patient deal constructively with his own problems? What capacities must he have acquired to be able to do so?" (Horney, p. 111).

Horney (1946b) contributes additional criteria for termination. Has the patient clarified his goals in life? Does the patient have a clear recognition of his own values? The patient needs to know in what direction he wants to develop. If his unhealthy goal is, for example, is vindictive triumph over others, he would want to become more efficient and destructive, certainly not a desirable therapy goal. This type of character disorder would not care to discover his incapacity for love. The patient must see himself as he is and could be instead of trying to establish an idealized, superior self involving the search for glory. The patient has hope and has overcome his "I can't" attitude. The patient has significantly reduced making others responsible for his difficulty. The patient has accepted that "heaven and hell" are within himself. The patient evidences a greater desire to work on himself. The patient shows a greater capability of observing his self outside of therapy. He is also more cooperative with the therapist in doing the work required of therapy.

In her paper "Pride and Self-Hatred" (1947), Horney presents the necessary stages for change. Without these stages existing in the patient, change will not take place, goals will not be reached, and therapy may end badly. She (Horney, p. 131) writes that awareness is required in the patient of what he is doing to himself as a person. Awareness has to be of a certain quality. It should not merely be an intellectual exaltation leading nowhere. Nor should it take the form of self-reproaches or seeing the conflict and figuring out ways to get around it.

Seeing consequences in our behavior is invaluable. Horney notes that viewing consequences may attract the patient's self-interest, but if that self-interest is in the service of self-hatred there will be little constructive change.

What has to happen for the patient after awareness? According to Horney (1947), the patient must retake his externalizations. He has to realize that it is not others' "shoulds," entitlements, or searches for glory, but his own claims and "shoulds." He has to view the problems as his own. He must persistently reevaluate his values. "To see the real values in life does away with cynicism and this goes on through the analysis" (Horney, p. 131). The patient will no longer see his need to retaliate as strength.

The patient progresses toward termination when he then can reevaluate his assets, see his true strength, and dispense with his self-hatred. His relationship with others improves. There is less sarcasm and anger. However, there are some patients who still balk at change unless they really hit bottom or see their life as a "sink or swim" choice. As Horney (1947, p. 132) puts it, the "Patient must face his own neurotic drives and see that he can't get well unless neurotic drives are given up. This is iron-clad psychological law that the patient must accept if he is to get well."

Horney (1947, pp. 132–133) counsels an important approach to a patient's despair and impasse. She suggests that the therapist see it as a riddle which requires thinking as to how it can be overcome. Horney (pp. 132–133) states:

> Then the next time the patient starts to see some things concretely and is much more constructive. Here is a fault, but the fault is not an all-prevailing poison gas. He hits the depths of despair and then starts to come up out of it.

With regard to the aims of the self, the patient's greater self-realization, along with constructive changes, directs him to become real without the influence of pride, hurt, or neurotic solutions. He sees others as they are, and does not misinterpret their motives or actions by externalizations or exploit them. He is more able to enjoy his work for its own sake and not as a path to glory. His increased self-realization "means that the person accepts his place in the world, with its attendant responsibility, and is aware of the broader issues" (Horney, 1956c, p. 177).

Boigon (1965), a Horneyan analyst, contributes to Horney's observation regarding the end of therapy by pointing out that it is difficult to evaluate positive change if the judgment is based on a reduction of the patient's anxiety. It is true that paradoxically the anxiety level of a patient may temporarily rise as he becomes more aware of the intensity of his self-hate and its consequences. I have found that expansive and narcissistic patients who begin to recognize how impaired their lives have been because of their character pathology develop increased anxiety. But Boigon notes that the increased anxiety of the character disorder as a consequence of change may not pose a treatment problem as long as it is not overwhelming. Neither can we depend on lessened symptoms, since they temporarily decrease during a forward movement but hopefully temporarily increase when the patient momentarily regresses. What about greater adaptation as a criteria? Not good, according to Boigon, since it may just mean more compulsive conformity. We have to distinguish between greater interpersonal freedom that is healthy, such as, greater capacity for empathy, concern, lessened narcissism, greater sense of appropriate responsibility, and lessened morbid dependency. Similarly, increased assertion may turn out to be aggression; withdrawal may be revealed as a retreat into phobic anxiety, not a retreat to increase a healthy consolidation of the real self. The patient's knowledge of himself must not remain an intellectual knowledge of himself but an emotional experience. Basically, the patient is ready for termination when he is more certain that he is the author of his fate. It is clear to him that it is not chance or the persecution of others that determines his destiny.

According to Horney (1949, p. 156), the mentally healthy individual can regret deeply what he has or has not accomplished but does not condemn himself. He is matter-of-fact and truthful with himself rather than blaming others. He does not assume too much or too little responsibility for making others happy. He does not have grandiose "shoulds" fostering guilt (Horney, p. 155). He can cope constructively with his problems.

The criteria for termination are, of course, ideals. All of them may not be realized toward the end of treatment but they also embody goals that the therapist needs to keep in mind. Some aims have already been mentioned.

Toward the end of therapy, the patient has clarified his goals and has a clearer recognition of his own values. He now knows in what direction he wishes to develop. He has discovered and laid to rest pathological goals such as vindictiveness, as with the patient, Bob, who took pride in his tenacious vindictiveness and relished his continued expression of it. The patient now knows or has a clearer idea of who he is and could be, instead of trying to establish his idealized self and promote his doomed search for glory. He has reduced his "I can not" attitudes and replaced them with realizable "I possibly can," or "I will at least give it my best shot."

When I first entered the field of psychotherapy, I was told by a supervisor not to expect gratitude from my patients when treatment had been successfully concluded. Nonetheless, it is a paradox that one of the criteria of successful therapy I have found is that the patient can now express gratitude more readily to family, friends, colleagues, and even to his therapist.

FINAL THOUGHTS

It is only fitting that this chapter end with the final thoughts of Karen Horney on the technique of psychotherapy in her last major work, "Neurosis and Human Growth" (1950a). Toward the end of the book she, in her usually lucid style, presented her major therapy ideas in the chapter "The Road of Psychoanalytic Therapy" (pp. 333–365).

To aid the patient, Horney suggests that the therapist help the patient get in touch with his real self. She suggests that the therapist encourage the patient to probe emotionally "Who am I?"

Horney (1950a, pp. 350–351) is convinced that "Only when the patient has become interested in the question 'Who am I' will the analyst more actively try to bring to his awareness how little he does know or care about his real feelings, wishes or beliefs."

A patient, wanting to be liberated from the problem of "Who am I?" and "What do I want to be?" and more specifically excessive compliance, gives Horney (1950a, pp. 351–352) the opportunity to demonstrate how the problem can be handled. Specific questions can be raised such as "Is compliance a function of having to run away from conflict with another, minimizing the value of his time or pridefully expecting of himself that he can accomplish everything?" Horney (p. 351) suggests that the analyst ask the patient "Has it never occurred to you to consult yourself what you want or deem right?" The patient, Horney advises, should be urged to try self-analysis in between therapy sessions. The therapist should also hold before the patient the good consequences of reducing his problem of excessive compliance, namely: being less anxious with others, less dependent on them, and better able to have a closer, equal, and sympathetic attitude for them.

Commenting about pathology in general, Horney (1950a, p. 363) writes "The neurotic is after all a magician living by his magic powers. Any step toward self-realization means relinquishing these powers and living by his existing resources. But as he realizes that he can in fact live without such illusions, and even live better without them, he gains faith in himself." And she (Horney, p. 377) observed that

> Man under the pressure of inner distress reaches out for the ultimate and the infinite which—though his limits are not fixed—it is not given to him to reach; and in this very process he destroys himself, shifting his very best drive for self-realization to the actualization of his idealized image and thereby wasting the potentialities he actually possesses [italics added].

12 Applying Horneyan Concepts Today

Probably 90% of patients in individual or couples therapy are seen nationwide on a once-per-week basis. Given this brief therapeutic encounter and the senseless managed care restrictions (e.g., 20 sessions permitted per year and a precise prediction when therapy will end), the patient's problems lend themselves more readily to Horney's concepts. Her ideas are presented in experience-near, closer to consciousness, level of awareness. Consequently, patients in most instances easily relate to interpretation couched in Horney's language. Paralleling the patient's relatively easy acceptance of Horneyan interventions, when I taught abnormal psychology many of my college students confessed that they saw themselves significantly more in her writings than in any other assigned psychoanalytic exposition. The working alliance is also strengthened more effectively when the patient feels understood through the application of Horneyan concepts.

Seeing patients for only one session during the week is much more difficult than psychoanalysis. It is especially difficult when one carries 30 or more patients coming one time per week. As Harold Kelman (1945) observed, once-per-week session therapy makes great demands on the therapist's energy and mental acuity. Still, the patient's progress depends ultimately on his or her motivation and it is possible that a poorly motivated patient in psychoanalysis will not do as well as one in psychotherapy who has good self-reflective capacities and a powerful motivation to grow.

In his book *Ego and Self in Weekly Psychotherapy*, Bocknek (1992) delineates various features of once-per-week psychotherapy. He thinks that weekly therapy dilutes interpretations, transference, and many other important properties of dynamic psychotherapy. Resistances become harder to deal with and a potential source of useful information is limited.

Stimulating the increasing popularity of weekly psychotherapy is the reality that the public, according to Bocknek (1992, p. 1), "has been disabused of the idyllic fantasies that once evoked of 'permanent cure' and total personality reorganization." They no longer believe that psychoanalysis individuals become paragons of mental health or that frequent (3 or more weekly sessions) necessarily guarantee greater or quicker cures. Nevertheless, he asserts that the growth of psychoanalytic understanding may also advance the effectiveness of weekly therapy. Clinical experience has convinced me that going back more vigorously to Karen Horney's insights and applying them to a greater extent to the treatment of character pathology would also further the capability of treatment.

When reading both the criticisms of Horney and praise of her ideas it is worth keeping in mind the following commentary by Ford and Urban (1965, p. 482) on Karen Horney and her system of psychotherapy:

> It is typical of reviewers to call attention to the various lapses and inconsistencies in her descriptive propositions and to criticize the ambiguity of definition in some of her concepts. These contrasts among the views of Karen Horney's work is somewhat analogous to the fate of a Broadway play which enjoys an extended run in the face of negative reviews by the drama critics. It seems likely in such an instance that despite formal lacks of one kind or another, there is much in the production that viewers can find of value, and which they can put to some good use.

CRITIQUE

Horney states that character disorder originates in part from cultural elements and distortions in interpersonal relationships. Specific cultural factors may determine an emphasis on certain character traits, such as aggressive competitiveness in relationships, work, love, or penis envy in women (i.e., the penis becomes symbolic of the male's superior power in our culture). Horney saw the envy not as part of a psychosexual biological inheritance but as the outcome of women's perception of the male's dominance in almost every sphere of life, the result of women's internalization of cultural male chauvinism.

With regard to the impact of culture on the formation of character disorder, Horney can be criticized on the grounds that she does not work out specifically how cultural elements or contradictory societal factors modify and/or create basic anxiety and the character disorder. She does not clarify enough how our culture impairs the character disorder's functioning.

Horney rejected Freud's instinct theory and the theory that behavior is directed by sexual and aggressive drives. She saw aggression as caused by frustration of fundamental needs for love, safety, security, and reduction of anxiety.

Rejecting instinctual sexual and aggressive drives, Horney can be criticized for neglecting their powerful, complex, biological contribution to the formation of the final character structure. Take, for example, Horney's moving toward people or compliant character structure disorder. The compliant patient's aggressive urges (*temperamentally enhanced*) may have been so discouraged and made anxiety-ridden during childhood that, as an adult, any success of the patient is perceived by him as an assault or forbidden aggressive rivalry with a competitor (e.g., parent or sibling).

Character disorders, Horney found, always have basic anxiety as their cornerstone. The helplessness or basic anxiety of the child leaves him or her vulnerable, with a conviction of being isolated and helpless in a possibly cruel world.

Horney's emphasis on basic anxiety derived from childhood helplessness and insecurity seems in part correct. But aside from basic anxiety in childhood, there is also pleasure in reduction of tension, and this gratification may determine the seemingly irrational, childish style of the character disorder. Horney does not address the clinical finding that anxiety can be further subdivided into diverse forms. The anxiety can be, for example, of loss of a body part such as hair, of a valued relationship, of a virtue, or of annihilation of the self. Not discussed by Horney in detail are the ingredients in the real self that determine how well an individual handles basic anxiety or pleasure-driven urges.

Horney asserted that people have the ability as well as the desire to evolve into reasonable human beings. An individual, she felt, can change and go on changing as long as he lives. Inherent in man is a desire to fulfill his given potentialities, a drive for self-realization.

However, does a character disorder inevitably have a frozen, healthy, embryonic real self waiting to be unleashed during the therapeutic disillusionment phase followed by the constructive process? Clinical experience says sometimes "yes" and occasionally "no." the drive for completion of healthy potentialities may be so totally damaged that the real self may never emerge. The real self may not see the light of day, for example, when huge blockages and/or safety measure are too powerful to overcome or reduce, such as massive pride in a character disorder solution.

Horney found that there is a need to value oneself and to be valued. Poor self-esteem is a consequence of either under- or over-valuation of the self. This leads to a specific idealized image by way of compensation.

On the other hand, with regard to self-esteem, some narcissistic character disorders may value themselves so highly that their self-esteem seldom falters. Indeed, progress in therapy is measured when they first register a modicum of discontent with their conceited, self-righteous idealized image.

Horney defined conflict broadly, seeing it as either a juxtaposition of the real self versus the idealized self, the real self versus the pride system, or the destructive forces versus the constructive urges. While this division is valuable at times, Horney neglected other important conflicts. To name a few, they are conflicts between the real self of the character disorder and the real self of another individual; conflicts between a strong claim and the same claim but weaker; passivity versus activity; masculinity versus femininity; idealized image versus another idealized image within the same individual; a particular "should" opposed to another "should" within the same individual or in opposition to another person; a malignant internalization of a parental image versus another parental composite.

The treatment of the present in therapy, Horney observed, is immeasurably more effective than the focus on the past. Cognitive therapists embrace this same finding.

Horney did consider the past as important in determining the char-acter structure. In her model it was more a matter of emphasis than total neglect. In any case once-per-week psychotherapy almost mandates a fo-cus on present events in the life of the patient. There just is not enough time to explore the patient's childhood in detail.

Horney's de-emphasis on the past may slight to a degree the possible effective, emotional impact on a patient's progress. Furthermore, on oc-casion, a foray into a patient's past can uncover significant events that the patient could not recall, thus furthering needed explanatory understand-ing or the value of an interpretation.

When called for, the therapist is free to borrow other useful concepts from different analytic schools to add details and dynamics neglected by Horney's theory. She, for example, omits the treatment of identifications, that is, whom the patient internalized. A knowledge of the clash of identifications within the self can prove useful in therapy. The Kleinian exposition (Solomon, 1995) of projective identification and introjec-tion may help explain many vexing transference and counter-transfer-ence issues.

13 A Horneyan Analysis of the Main Character in Brian Moore's Novel *The Statement*

In this chapter I apply Horney's theory of character structure to Pierre Brossard, the central protagonist in Brian Moore's novel, (1996) *The Statement*. Pierre Brossard, a Vichy, Nazi collaborator and murderer of Jews, is eluding pursuers whom he mistakenly believes are Jewish. Brossard, within Horney's model, clearly falls within the "moving against others" type. Karen Horney's observations with regard to the "moving against others" character disorder clarify Brossard's psychic functioning in terms of his claims, pride, "should," self-hate, and idealized image. The role of his self-hate in ultimately impairing his cunning is shown in his ignoring evidence that would have saved his life.

Before I apply Horney's insights to this powerful novel, we can be grateful to Paris (1974), who assiduously demonstrated how well the Horneyan model exposed the nuances of character structure in great literature in general. In a later biography of Horney, Paris (1994, pp. 247–249) steers us to other authors who also have fruitfully applied the Horneyan model to various character types in literature, such as the self-effacing, arrogant-vindictive, perfectionistic, narcissistic, and detached types. Biographers (Paris, 1994, p. 250) too have looked at their subject through the prism of Horney's concepts and profited from an enhanced understanding of the subject's psychic structure. As Paris (1994, p. 226) points out, Horney's approach has been especially useful to psychohistorians since it does not rely on a subject's early childhood history, which is often not available to a biographer.

SUMMARY OF THE BOOK

Brian Moore's slender novel can serve as an excellent illustration of the value of applying Horney's ideas of character structure, but first I shall give a brief summary of the book. The chief protagonist is Brossard, a 70-year-old Vichy, Nazi collaborator, thief, and murderer. When we first meet him he is living in a monastery in France, protected by a priest who is sympathetic to him as supposedly a repentant sinner. Apparently for some priests, the passport to protection and shelter for someone with Brossard's history of anti-Semitism and murder of Jews is merely his participation in a confession. All sins are then supposedly forgiven. Pierre Brossard is being pursued by assassins disguised as Jews whom he outfoxes and kills. Ironically, the group employing the assassins are the very same individuals in high political circles who collaborated with the Vichy Nazi regime. They wish to do away with Brossard to protect themselves from the consequences of a military and clerical investigation. Until now this same group and another group, the Chevaliers, have financially supported and protected Brossard for 44 years as he successfully eluded proper punishment for his crimes against humanity. Brossard is lulled into a false sense of security by his long-term supporters and is done in by someone he trusts. As he dies, he sees the Jews he has murdered as if in a courtroom and realizes to his horror that his false piety will not prevent his being properly punished for his sins in the next world.

INTERPRETATION

Pierre Brossard appears to be an excellent example of an individual within the "moving against others" category described so well by Horney's book *Our Inner Conflicts* (1945). He is filled with anger. He, for example, refers to his wife as a "Poor bitch, what use was she to anyone now?" (Moore, 1996, p. 114). He loved executions. They were a form of war. The enemy was cornered and in his power. He was God. He gave the order: "He and LeGrand walked down the line, giving the coup de grace, a bullet in the back of the neck" (p. 117). Thus Brossard gleefully kills 14 Jews.

Horney (1945) points out that the "moving against others" type is characterized by "a callous pursuit of self-interest . . . an outright exercise of power" (p. 64). When Brossard murders the Jews he thinks "It was the moment of joy, the moment of power I am God. I am God" (p. 116). Toward Bobi, his former wife Nicole's cherished old, blind dog, Brossard "took aim and neatly kicked Bobi in the throat. The dog choked, then howled" (p. 151).

What are Brossard's values? Horney (1945) describes them well. "His set of values is built around the philosophy of the jungle. Might makes right. Away with humanness and mercy" (pp. 68–69). Horney points out that "his sadistic dealings with others provide him with a feeling of strength and pride which reinforce his unconscious feeling of omnipotence" (p. 207). Brossard, for example, feels like God when he murders the helpless Jews. Horney further contributes an insight into Brossard's character when she notes that "He . . . may consciously experience elation at being able to do with others as he pleases" (p. 207).

Brossard wants to die in a state of grace. He feels entitled, a claim, to be free of any sin since he is heard in confession by a priest who can give him words of absolution. He is convinced that "Confession was the greatest sacrament of the Church, a passport out of the flames of hell" (Moore, 1996, p. 58).

Although one part of Brossard feels that he should be absolved through confession, another part has doubts. He recognizes that his whole life has been an imposture. He has a fleeting insight that he is lying even when he is telling the truth. However, Brossard quickly credits himself with virtue and pride in that virtue for just seeking out a confessor under the most dangerous conditions. His defense machinery kicks in very easily to halt any eruption of guilt and/or basic anxiety.

Brossard bears out Horney's astute observation that "Those neurotics who have entrenched themselves in a shell of self-righteousness have so silenced all self-accusations that nothing reaches awareness" (1950, pp. 115–116), and

> He may have an equally strong interest in not perceiving *contradictory values* co-existing in him. Quite literally, he may utterly fail to see that he tolerates and even cherishes in himself two sets of values, both conscious, which are mutually contradictory (Horney, p. 180).

In the case of Brossard, he demonstrates a pretense of piety and consistent sadism.

Brossard is a keen observer of behavior and is able to accurately discern from a priest's slightest gesture, tone, and facial expression whether he will or will not aid him. Yet his hatred of Jews is so great that he never puts "two and two" together to come up with the plausible hypothesis that it is not the vengeful Jews who are trying to persistently assassinate him. He does not use the obvious fact that the assassin's knowledge of his itinerary indicates that possibly his supposed protectors want him dead. In a sense, his self-hate surfaces here and manifests itself through a destructive impairment of his ordinarily razor-sharp mind, and he falls prey to his protectors. His demise reflects the African proverb that it is on the path that you fear the least that the wild beast strikes.

In conclusion, I have applied Horney's model of character pathology to the main character, Pierre Brossard, in Brian Moore's novel (1996), *The Statement*. Brossard falls clearly within the interpersonal type, "moving against others." He is, more specifically, an egocentric, sadistic, ruthless, cunning man who is very adroit at manipulating others and anticipating any threat to him. His chief claim is to be able to hurt others with impunity. His main "should" is one where he can be assured of entering heaven as a cleansed sinner despite his horrific crimes against humanity. He also feels a neurotic pride in his participation as a Nazi collaborator in the Vichy regime. His self-hate emerges in the impaired functioning of his ordinarily superior anticipatory judgment. Ultimately, his impaired cognitive function blinds him fatally to the true employers of the assassins sent to murder him. As he dies he realizes to his horror that his pretense of piety is not going to admit him to the glory of God's forgiving, loving embrace. Instead, the Jews he murdered will render a well-deserved verdict and penalty that will send him eternally to hell's nether regions.

Brossard wanted glory and believed he had found it in a moment of sadistic power, but, as Horney states, "the easy way to infinite glory is inevitably also the way to an inner hell of self-contempt and self-torment. By taking this road, the individual is in fact losing his soul—his real self" (1950a, p. 39).

References

American Psychiatric Association. (1994). *DSM-IV*. Washington, DC: Author.

Bocknek, G. (1992). *Ego and self in weekly psychotherapy.*New York: International Universities Press.

Boigon, M., et al. (1965). What leads to basic change in psychoanalytic theory. *American Journal of Psychoanalysis, 25,* 129–141.

Cameron, D. E. (1954). Karen Horney: A pioneer in the science of human relations. *American Journal of Psychoanalysis, 14,* 19–29.

Connelly, M. (2002). *Bones.* New York: Little Brown.

Ellis, A. (1963). *Reason and emotion in psychotherapy.* New York: Lyle Stuart.

Ford, H. D., & Urban, H. B. (1965). *Systems of psychotherapy.* New York: John Wiley and Sons.

Freud, A. (1946). *The ego and the mechanisms of defense.* London: Hogarth Press.

Horney, K. (1917). The technique of psychoanalytic therapy. *American Journal of Psychoanalysis, 28,* 3–12. In Paris, B. J. (Ed.). (1999). *Karen Horney: The therapeutic process* (pp. 11–23). New Haven, CT: Yale University Press.

Horney, K. (1935a). Conceptions and misconceptions of the analytic method. *Journal of Nervous and Mental Disease, 81,* 399–410. In Paris, B. J. (Ed.). (1999). *Karen Horney: The therapeutic process* (pp. 32–44). New Haven, CT: Yale University Press.

Horney, K. (1935b). On difficulties in dealing with the transference. *The News-Letter of the American Association of Psychiatric Social Workers, 5*(2), 1 5. In Paris, B. J. (Ed.). (1999). *Karen Horney: The therapeutic process* (pp. 52–56). New Haven, CT: Yale University Press.

Horney, K. (1936). The problem of the negative therapeutic reaction. *Psychoanalytic Quarterly, 5,* 29–44. In Paris, B. J. (Ed.). (1999). *Karen Horney: The therapeutic process* (pp. 59–71). New Haven, CT: Yale University Press.

Horney, K. (1937). *The neurotic personality of our time*. New York: W. W. Norton.

Horney, K. (1939). *New ways in psychoanalysis*. New York: W. W. Norton.

Horney, K. (1942). *Self-analysis*. New York: W. W. Norton.

Horney, K. (1945). *Our inner conflicts*. New York: W. W. Norton.

Horney, K. (1946a). Are you considering psychoanalysis? In Paris, B. J. (Ed.). (1999). *Karen Horney: The therapeutic process* (pp. 97–109). New Haven, CT: Yale University Press.

Horney, K. (1946b) How do you progress after analysis?" In Paris, B. J. (Ed.). (1999). *Karen Horney: The therapeutic process* (pp. 110–122). New Haven, CT: Yale University Press.

Horney, K. (1947). Pride and self-hatred. In Paris, B. J. (Ed.). (1999). *Karen Horney: The therapeutic process* (pp. 126–133). New Haven, CT: Yale University Press.

Horney, K. (1949). Finding the real self: A letter with a foreword by Karen Horney. *American Journal of Psychoanalysis, 9*, 3–7. In Paris, B. J. (Ed.). (1999). *Karen Horney: The therapeutic process* (pp. 134–142). New Haven, CT: Yale University Press.

Horney, K. (1950a). *Neurosis and human growth: The struggle toward self-realization*. New York: W. W. Norton.

Horney, K. (1950b). Psychotherapy. Talk given by Karen Horney at the Institute of Living in New York City. *Digest of Neurology and Psychiatry, 18*, 278. In Paris, B. J. (Ed.). (1999). *Karen Horney: The therapeutic process* (pp. 156–157). New Haven, CT: Yale University Press.

Horney, K. (1956a). Interpretations (reconstructed by Ralph Slater). *American Journal of Psychoanalysis, 16*, 118–124. In Paris, B. J. (Ed.). (1999). *Karen Horney: The therapeutic process* (pp. 206–214). New Haven, CT: Yale University Press.

Horney, K. (1956b). Understanding the patient as the basis of all technique (compiled by Emy A. Metzger from lectures on psychoanalytic technique given by Karen Horney at the American Institute for Psychoanalysis during 1946, 1950, 1951, & 1952). *American Journal of Psychoanalysis, 16*, 26–31. In Paris, B. J. (Ed.). (1999). *Karen Horney: The therapeutic process* (pp. 198–205). New Haven, CT: Yale University Press.

Horney, K. (1956c). Aims of psychoanalytic therapy (reconstructed by Ralph Slater). *American Journal of Psychoanalysis, 16*, 118–124. In Paris, B. J. (Ed). (1999). *Karen Horney: The therapeutic process* (pp. 175–177). New Haven, CT: Yale University Press.

Horney, K. (1957a). The analyst's personal equation (compiled by Louis A. Azorin from lectures on psychoanalytic technique given by Karen Horney at the American Institute for Psychoanalysis during 1946, 1950, 1951, &

1952). *American Journal of Psychoanalysis, 16*, 118–124. In Paris, B. J. (Ed.). (1999). *Karen Horney: The therapeutic process* (pp. 191–197). New Haven, CT: Yale University Press.

Horney, K. (1957b). The initial interview, part 1 (compiled by Morton B. Cantor from lectures on psychoanalytic technique given by Karen Horney at the American Institute for Psychoanalysis during 1946, 1950, 1951, & 1952). *American Journal of Psychoanalysis, 17*, 39–44. In Paris, B. J. (Ed.). (1999). *Karen Horney: The therapeutic process* (pp. 178–185). New Haven, CT: Yale University Press.

Horney, K. (1958). Dreams, part 1: Theoretical considerations (compiled by Wanda Willig from lectures on psychoanalytic technique given by Karen Horney at the American Institute for Psychoanalysis). *American Journal of Psychoanalysis, 18*, 127–231. In Paris, B. J. (Ed.). (1999). *Karen Horney: The therapeutic process* (pp. 222–231). New Haven, CT: Yale University Press.

Horney, K. (1960). Evaluation of change (compiled by Ralph Slater from lectures given during 1952 and 1953 by Karen Horney at the American Institute for Psychoanalysis). *American Journal of Psychoanalysis, 20*, 200. In Paris, B. J. (Ed.). (1999). *Karen Horney: The therapeutic process* (pp. 242–247). New Haven, CT: Yale University Press.

Horney, K. (1967). *Feminine psychology*. Kelman, H. (Ed.). New York: W. W. Norton.

Horney, K. (1987). *Final lectures*. Ingram, D. H. (Ed.). New York: W. W. Norton.

Horney, K. (1999). *The therapeutic process*. Paris, B. J. (Ed.). New Haven, CT: Yale University Press.

Horney, K. (2000). *The unknown Karen Horney: Essays on gender, culture, and psychoanalysis*. Paris, B. J. (Ed.). New Haven, CT: Yale University Press.

Ivimey, M. (1950). Childhood memories. *American Journal of Psychoanalysis, 10*, 38–47.

Kaiser, H. (1965). The problem of responsibility in psychotherapy. In L. B. Fierman (Ed.), *Effective psychotherapy: The contributions of Hellmuth Kaiser*. New York: Free Press.

Kelman, H. (1945). Analysis once a week. *American Journal of Psychoanalysis, 5*, 16–87.

Klein, M. (1975). An obsessional neurosis in a six-year old girl. In *The writings of Melanie Klein* (vol. II, pp. 35–57). London: Hogarth Press.

Klein, M. (1975). Envy and gratitude. In *The writings of Melanie Klein* (vol. III, pp. 176–235). London: Hogarth.

Kohut, H. (1971). *The analysis of the self*. New York: International Universities Press.

Kohut, H. (1977). *The restoration of the self*. New York: International Universities Press.

Landman, L. (1959). Dynamics of hostility. *American Journal of Psychoanalysis, 19*, 13–18.

Lasch, C. (1979). *The culture of narcissism: American life in an age of diminishing expectations*. New York: W. W. Norton.

Mahler, M. S., Pine, F., & Bergman, A. (1975). *The psychological birth of the human infant: Symbiosis and individuation*. New York: Basic Books.

Manrique, J. F. D. (1984). Hope as a means of therapy in the work of Karen Horney. *American Journal of Psychoanalysis, 44*, 301–331.

Martin, A. R. (1966). Emphasis on the healthy aspects of the patient in psycho-analysis. *American Journal of Psychoanalysis, 26*, 201–206.

Martin, A. R. (1978). Adapting psychoanalytic procedure to the uniqueness of the individual. *American Journal of Psychoanalysis, 38*, 99–110.

Miller, F. (1977). Differential diagnostic considerations in neurosis and character disorder. *American Journal of Psychoanalysis, 37*, 309–315.

Moore, B. (1996). *The statement*. New York: Dutton.

Paris, B. J. (1974). *A psychological approach to fiction: Studies on Thackeray, Stendhal, George Eliot, Dostoevsky, and Conrad*. Bloomington: Indiana University Press.

Paris, B. J. (1994). *Karen Horney: A psychoanalyst's search for self-understanding*. New Haven, CT: Yale University Press.

Passoni, J. (1952). Constructive and obstructive forces in psychoanalysis. *American Journal of Psychoanalysis, 21*, 74–77.

Paul, H. A. (1989). Karen Horney's theory of self. In D. W. Detrick & S. P. Detrick (Eds.), *Self psychology: Comparisons and contrasts*. Hillsdale, NJ: Analytic Press.

Quinn, S. (1987). *A mind of her own: The life of Karen Horney*. New York: Summit.

Reich, W. (1933). *Character analysis* (Theodore Wolfe, Trans.). Rangely, ME: Orgone Institute Press.

Rodale, J. M. (1978). *The synonym finder*. Emmaus, PA: Rodale Press.

Rubins, J. L. (1978). *Karen Horney: Gentle rebel of psychoanalysis*. New York: Dial Press.

Seligman, M. E. P. (1991). *Learned optimism*. New York: W. W. Norton.

Smith, S. (1977). The golden fantasy: A regressive reaction to separation anxiety. *International Journal of Psychoanalysis, 58*, 311–324.

Solomon, I. (1985). On feeling hopeless. *Psychoanalytic Review, 72*, 55–69. In Solomon, I. (1992). *The encyclopedia of evolving techniques in dynamic Psychotherapy* (pp. 127–137). Northvale, NJ: Jason Aronson.

Solomon, I. (1995). *A primer of Kleinian therapy*. Northvale, NJ: Jason Aronson.

Sterba, R. F. (1953). Clinical and therapeutic aspects of character resistance. *Psychoanalytic Quarterly, 22*, 1–20.

Symonds, M. (1970). Marital disharmony and character structure. *American Journal of Psychoanalysis, 30*, 73–80.

Tarachow, S. (1963). *An introduction to psychotherapy*. New York: International Universities Press.

Van Bark, B. (1959). Dynamics of hostility: A panel. *American Journal of Psychoanalysis, 19*, 21–27.

Ward, H. P. (1972). Aspects of shame in analysis. *American Journal of Psychoanalysis, 32*, 62–73.

Wassell, B. (1955). The analytic relationship. *American Journal of Psychoanalysis, 15*, 22–30.

Wenkart, A. (1955). Self-acceptance. *American Journal of Psychoanalysis, 15*, 135–143.

Whitman, W. (1861). *Leaves of grass*. Philadelphia: David McKay.

Winnicott, D. W. (1974). Fear of breakdown. *International Journal of Psychoanalysis, 1*, 103–107.

Yalom, D. I. (2002). *The gift of therapy: An open letter to a generation of therapists and their patients*. New York: Harper Collins.

Glossary of Horneyan Terms

Alienation from the self is being cut off from one's feelings, an unwillingness to grow, not being in the driver's seat, unaware of who we really are and what we are doing, unreflective.

Automatic controls are feelings and impulses automatically checked to avoid disintegration of the self. Automatic control may be accompanied by pride, depicting the control as dignity.

Blockages (resistances) are manifestations such as of forces that the patient mobilizes to fight off healthy change or to preserve the familiar or status quo. Various defensive maneuvers are employed. Secret claims are tenaciously held and appear in treatment. Blockages impede progress but paradoxically provide invaluable insights into neurotic character functioning.

Character trends are moving toward, against, and away from people.

Claims are entitlements to special concern, attention, and deference; a conviction that whatever the patient thinks, feels, or does will not have any negative consequences. The frustration of a wish or need is experienced as a personal offense against the patient.

Compartmentalization (psychic fragmentation) is when the patient has no feeling for himself as a whole individual. He disconnects by only registering an interpretation or new insight intellectually. There may be blindness to an obvious cause and effect. Existing contradictions are not seen. Compartmentalization serves to maintain the status quo.

Conflicts occur between the real self and the pseudo-self, the opposition between the glorified self and the despised self or the true self. Conflicts may appear between expansiveness versus self-effacement, one claim versus another claim, "should" versus "should," pride versus pride, destructive forces in opposition to constructive forces, and the pride system opposing the true self.

Counter-transference appears when the therapist unconsciously misunderstands and/or misperceives and treats the patient in terms of his own idealized image, pride, claims, "shoulds." In short, the therapist's character disorder, if not regulated by his true self, colors his interventions and injects destructive elements into the treatment process.

Expansive solutions are employed by the patient in identification with his grandiose, idealized self. He has the conviction that every obstacle can be overcome. His main fear is helplessness and self-effacement. There is a pretense of being all-knowing. Narcissism, perfectionism, and arrogant-vindictiveness are usually present.

Externalization occurs when what is experienced internally is felt as existing between the self and the outside world. It is a way of preserving the idealized image by blaming others for one's limitations. It is also a means of dampening the inner conflict between self-destructive and constructive forces.

Hopelessness manifests its ugly head when the patient despairs of ever changing in a healthy manner, of ever freeing himself from his character pathology. Hopelessness must be addressed constantly if therapy is to succeed.

Idealized self (image) is a self-picture that drives the patient to believe that he can be or is perfect, omniscient, and omnipotent. The idealized self pushes for glory. The true self is held in contempt for being weak and inhibiting of the special accomplishments that can and/or will be obtained through the actualization of the idealized self.

Negative therapeutic reaction is a rapid regression of treatment and return of symptoms shortly after a constructive movement.

Pride (unhealthy) is present based on a glorified image of the self. Pride may be attached to unreal or unhealthy convictions, feelings, and thoughts, such as being a saint or sufferer. Unhealthy pride is always in the service of the idealized self.

Search for glory maintains in the patient a riveting, driven vision of an eventual magnificent, grandiose future. This future, it is thought, can be attained through the diligent expression of character trends, solutions, claims, "shoulds," prides, and, of course, the idealized image.

Self-hate manifests itself in the patient as self-accusations, self-contempt, self-frustrations, self-torments. self-destruction, self-indictments by pride and "should." The patient may feel like a fraud, lack self-compassion, embrace guilt, and be exquisitely vulnerable to anything that smacks of criticism.

"Shoulds" are powerful compulsions and inner dictates that are activated within the patient to achieve grandiose success and glory. "Shoulds" are inevitably in the service of a neurotic character solution and/or an idealized image.

Solutions are neurotic, comprehensive answers that the character disorder develops to satisfy compulsively all his inner needs, conflicts, claims, and so forth.

Streamlining is a pattern of rigidly subduing forever one's self and functioning as another self, such as evolving as a proud self against a depressed self.

Supremacy of the mind enables the patient to set up a dichotomy wherein the mind opposes the body's needs or combats constructive self-interest. The mind becomes detached, a mere onlooker of the self. There is little interest in valuable insights related to the patient's life. Supremacy of the mind can lead to sadistically finding fault either with others or with one's self.

Transference is a function of the neurotic character structure that compels the patient to misperceive the therapist in terms of claims, "shoulds," trends, and so forth.

True self is sometimes referred to by Karen Horney as the real self. It is the alive part of our self, that part that assumes responsibility for an active role in deciding and giving inner independence and a healthy desire to grow.

Working alliance is the cooperation between the empathic, competent genuine true self of the therapist with that part of the patient's intact self that seeks to change and grow. It is characterized by the ongoing dedicated, constructive friendliness of the therapist to the patient.

Author Index

Subject Index